USING GROUNDED THEORY RESEARCH METHODS

A Guide for the Health and Social Sciences

Cheryl Tatano Beck

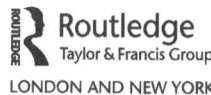 Routledge
Taylor & Francis Group

LONDON AND NEW YORK

Designed cover image: Shutterstock

First published 2026
by Routledge
4 Park Square, Milton Park, Abingdon, Oxon OX14 4RN

and by Routledge
605 Third Avenue, New York, NY 10158

Routledge is an imprint of the Taylor & Francis Group, an informa business

British Library Cataloguing-in-Publication Data
A catalogue record for this book is available from the British Library

Library of Congress Cataloging-in-Publication Data
Names: Beck, Cheryl Tatano author
Title: Using grounded theory research methods / Cheryl Tatano Beck.
Description: Abingdon, Oxon ; New York, NY : Routledge, 2026. | Includes bibliographical references and index.
Identifiers: LCCN 2025023672 (print) | LCCN 2025023673 (ebook) | ISBN 9781032695556 hardback | ISBN 9781032695549 paperback | ISBN 9781032695563 ebook
Subjects: LCSH: Grounded theory | Qualitative research--Methodology
Classification: LCC H61.24 .B43 2026 (print) | LCC H61.24 (ebook) | DDC 001.4/2--dc23/eng/20250721
LC record available at https://lccn.loc.gov/2025023672
LC ebook record available at https://lccn.loc.gov/2025023673

ISBN: 978-1-032-69555-6 (hbk)
ISBN: 978-1-032-69554-9 (pbk)
ISBN: 978-1-032-69556-3 (ebk)

DOI: 10.4324/9781032695563

Typeset in Sabon
by KnowledgeWorks Global Ltd.

USING GROUNDED THEORY RESEARCH METHODS

This practical text introduces and compares all the different varieties of grounded theory for researchers new to the methodology from across the health and social sciences. Grounded theory is a complex research methodology, further complicated by the existence of a number of different variations.

Method slurring is a common problem and this thoughtful textbook enables readers to understand and use grounded theory correctly, with chapters focusing on Barney Glaser's grounded theory, Anselm Strauss and Juliet Corbin's grounded theory, Leonard Schatzman and Barbara Bowers' dimensional analysis, Kathy Charmaz's constructivist grounded theory, and Adele Clarke's situational analysis. It includes a comparison of first- and second-generation grounded theory approaches and includes an interdisciplinary selection of examples. Each chapter includes tips for researchers, activities, and a summary highlighting the strengths and limitations of the grounded theory approach in question.

This text is an essential read for researchers with an interest in grounded theory or advanced students opting qualitative research methods courses.

Cheryl Tatano Beck is a distinguished professor at the School of Nursing, and has a joint appointment in the Department of Obstetrics and Gynecology at the School of Medicine, University of Connecticut, USA.

This book is dedicated to my loving family: My husband, Chuck, and children, Curt and Lisa. Words cannot express my appreciation for their continuous encouragement and support.

CONTENTS

PREFACE

In teaching qualitative research methods at the University of Connecticut for over 25 years at both the undergraduate and graduate levels, the qualitative design that students had the most difficult time grasping was grounded theory. I believe this is because it is the most complex design out of all the other qualitative designs such as narrative analysis or phenomenology. Three decades ago, grounded theorists were lamenting the methodological mistakes in published grounded theory studies (Baker et al., 1992; Becker, 1993; Wilson & Hutchinson, 1996). Wilson and Hutchinson warned researchers about muddling grounded theory methods while Baker et al. (1992) labeled this disturbing problem, method slurring. Researchers were mixing and matching different qualitative designs in one study. This corruption of methods in a study weakens its rigor and credibility. Thirty years later method slurring in grounded theory continues and led me to write an editorial for the *Journal of Obstetric, Gynecologic, and Neonatal Nursing* entitled, Avoiding potential pitfalls in qualitative research methods (Beck, 2022).

The aim of this proposed book is to help eradicate the decades long muddling of grounded theory methods. Part of this continuing eroding of correct grounded theory methods is that some researchers use published studies in top tier journals as templates for their own grounded theory studies. Using templates of methodologically weak grounded theory studies has perpetuated method slurring. An example of this method slurring can occur when researchers use some of Glaser's (1978) grounded theory methods and infiltrate these with some of Corbin and Strauss' (2015) methods in the same study.

Currently there is not a book published that compares and contrasts the methods of all the different grounded theory approaches. This book is cross-disciplinary. It is written for graduate students, faculty, and researchers from all disciplines where qualitative research is conducted. Examples of these disciplines include Nursing, Sociology, Psychology, Social Work, Medicine, Anthropology, Business, and Education. Professors who teach qualitative methodology courses, graduate students, junior faculty who are conducting a grounded theory study for the first time, and senior faculty who have not taken any qualitative methods courses that focused on grounded theory are all appropriate audiences for this book. Manuscript reviewers for journals and grant reviewers also need to understand the different versions of grounded theory in order to competently evaluate the rigor of a grant or manuscript using this complex qualitative methodology. Mixed methods research has definitely gained momentum in the last couple of decades. Quantitative researchers who are considering a mixed methods study are in need of qualitative methods textbooks, such as this one for grounded theory, to guide them through the qualitative strand which may not be their area of expertise.

This book has been a desire of mine since I started teaching PhD students qualitative research methodology courses at the University of Connecticut. What I wished for each semester as I was filling out my required textbook order form for my courses was one textbook that concentrated on a comparison of the different methodologies of grounded theory. I needed to piece together multiple readings on different grounded theory methodologies for my students. I hope by publishing this textbook other faculty and students will reap its benefits.

This is an exciting time in grounded theory with the wave of what is called the second generation of grounded theory approaches (Morse et al., 2021), which has evolved from Glaser and Strauss' (1967) original method. All the second-generation grounded theorists were former doctoral students of Glaser and Strauss. Second-generation grounded theory methods include Corbin and Strauss' grounded theory, dimensional analysis, situational analysis, and constructivist ground theory. Now with these new grounded theory approaches, the risk increases of method slurring if researchers are not educated about the differences in these methods. One version of grounded theory is not better than another. It is what fits best with the researcher, their philosophy, the research questions, and the population to be studied. Mixed method grounded theory, grounded theory with quantitative data, and formal grounded theory are also options for researchers. These approaches, however, are outside the purview of this book.

Since this book has a health and social sciences focus, I have included examples from these fields in most chapters to illustrate various methods. Periodically in the chapters there are boxes on tips for new researchers. Faculty, students, and qualitative researchers from across the globe hopefully will benefit from this book which has an international perspective. There are student exercises at the end of most chapters. For example, in one of the final chapters, students are directed to choose one of the grounded theory approaches described in this textbook and conduct an interdisciplinary search using various databases for grounded theory studies that used this approach. Students will then select one study from their search that is of interest to them and critique its methodology. Students can share their studies with the rest of the class. Another activity will be to have each student focus on their discipline. Using the primary database for their discipline for the past 5 years, such as ERIC for education, students can report back to the class on the number of published grounded theory studies in their discipline and which specific ground theory approach was used most often.

References

Baker, C., Wuest, J., & Stern, P. N. (1992). Method slurring: The grounded theory/phenomenology example. *Journal of Advanced Nursing, 17*(11), 1355–1360. https://doi.org/10.1111/j.1365-2648.1992.tb01859.x

Beck, C. T. (2022). Avoiding potential pitfalls in qualitative research methods. *Journal of Obstetric, Gynecologic, and Neonatal Nursing, 51*(5), 473–476. https://doi.org/10.1016/j.jogn.2022.08.002

Becker, P. H. (1993). Common pitfalls in published grounded theory research. *Qualitative Health Research, 3*(2), 254–260. https://doi.org/10.1177/104973239300300207

Corbin, J., & Strauss, A. (2015). *Basics of qualitative research: Techniques and procedures for developing grounded theory* (4th ed.). Sage.

Glaser, B. G. (1978). *Theoretical sensitivity: Advances in the methodology of grounded theory*. Sociology Press.

Glaser, B. G., & Strauss, A. (1967). *The discovery of grounded theory: Strategies for qualitative research*. Aldine de Gruyter.

Morse, J. M., Bowers, B. J., Charmaz, K., Clarke, A. E., Corbin, J., & Porr, C. J. (Eds.) (2021). *Developing grounded theory: The second generation revisited*. Routledge.

Wilson, H. S., & Hutchinson, S. A. (1996). Methodologic mistakes in grounded theory. *Nursing Research, 45*(2), 122–124.

ACKNOWLEDGMENTS

My sincere gratitude and thanks are extended to the staff at Routledge who have been tremendously helpful in bringing this project to completion.

Specifically, I am so grateful to Grace McInnes, Editor Health and Social Care, who took a chance on me years ago to publish my first book with Routledge. Now with her devoted support for my work, she has spearheaded my fourth book with Routledge. I could never have accomplished this without her expert guidance and encouragement over the years.

Also, I am so thankful to Madaline Cherry-Moreton who was the editorial assistant for my project. She was absolutely a delight to work with. No question of mine was too small or insignificant for her as she would immediately respond with her expert guidance.

In addition, I would like to extend my gratitude to the Production Team, namely the project manager, Saranya J., and copyeditor, Monika Kulshrestha, at KGL for their expert follow-through in the production process which was smooth and seamless.

My thanks are also extended to Dr. Carrie Morgan Eaton, my dear friend and fellow professor at the University of Connecticut, who put great effort into creating most of the artwork for this book. I would also like to recognize Madeleine Willett, an undergraduate nursing student at the University of Connecticut, who spent part of her summer helping with the first drafts of some of the figures.

My acknowledgment would not be complete without thanking my husband, Chuck, and children, Lisa and Curt, who provided ongoing support and encouragement throughout this and all my scholarly endeavors.

1

INTRODUCTION TO THE BOOK

This first chapter provides an overview of the book and its purpose. In this introductory chapter, a brief summary of what each of the other ten chapters covers is included.

Chapter 2 – And So It Began: Barney Glaser and Anselm Strauss' Grounded Theory

In this chapter how grounded theory began with Glaser and Strauss' (1967) book entitled *The Discovery of Grounded Theory: Strategies for Qualitative Research* is described. Their classic method of grounded theory is presented. Strauss and Glaser met at the University of California San Francisco (UCSF) School of Nursing, where the Dean had hired Strauss to teach in the PhD program. Strauss had received a large grant to study dying patients in hospitals and he recruited Glaser to join the faculty at UCSF and work with him on the grant. The development of their grounded theory method was an outcome of this grant.

Chapter 3 – Glaserian Grounded Theory

Glaser continued refining this method with his 1978 book entitled *Theoretical Sensitivity: Advances in the Methodology of Grounded Theory*. This became known as classic or Glaserian grounded theory, and is explained in this chapter. Glaser was a strong proponent of researchers continuing to modify their grounded theories. A grounded theory should not become stagnant. There are, however, few published grounded theory modifications. I have recently (Beck, 2023) published the third modification of my grounded theory of postpartum depression, Teetering on the Edge. This modification is described in the chapter as an illustration.

DOI: 10.4324/9781032695563-1

Chapter 4 – Straussian Grounded Theory

After the 1967 publication of *The Discovery of Grounded Theory: Strategies for Qualitative Research*, Strauss parted ways with Glaser to develop with Juliet Corbin, who completed a postdoctoral fellowship with him, what is known as Straussian grounded theory. Their grounded theory approach is presented in this chapter along with Corbin's modifications to their method after Strauss' death.

Chapter 5 – Leonard Schatzman and Barbara Bowers' Dimensional Analysis

In this chapter dimensional analysis, a second-generation grounded theory approach, is the focus. Leonard Schatzman (1991) developed dimensional analysis and later collaborated with Barbara Bowers, one of his former doctoral students (Bowers & Schatzman, 2009; 2021). Schatzman had been a PhD student of Strauss and then went on to become a colleague and publish with him. This grounded theory approach in addition to constant comparison of data, adds other analytic procedures. Schatzman took a broader approach to analysis of qualitative data than Strauss.

Chapter 6 – Adele Clarke's Situational Analysis

In this chapter Adele Clarke et al.'s (2018) second-generation grounded theory approach is front and center. In situational analysis the situation under study is the key unit of analysis. The researcher uses identified relational analyses as the researcher creates four types of analytic maps to help uncover the complexities of a specific situation: Situational maps, relational maps, social worlds/arenas maps, and positional maps.

Chapter 7 – Kathy Charmaz's Constructivist Grounded Theory

In reviewing recent databases, Charmaz's constructivist grounded theory is currently being used most often in published studies. Her second-generation modification of grounded theory is described in this chapter. Charmaz (2025) in her method stressed the researcher participates in co-constructing the data with the participants. She emphasized the reflexivity of the researcher throughout the research process.

Chapter 8 – Comparison of First- and Second-Generation Grounded Theory Approaches

This chapter covers the comparison of the methods of first- and second-generation grounded theory methods. One method is not better than the other one. What is most important is that whichever approach researchers choose, they pay meticulous attention to that method and are not guilty of continuing the slurring of methods.

Chapter 9 – Critiquing Grounded Theory Studies

Various frameworks are addressed in this chapter that have been published to aid in evaluating grounded theory studies. Glaser and Strauss, Glaser, Strauss and Corbin, and Charmaz all have included criteria that can be used to critique the rigor of a grounded theory study. Morse et al. (2021) also identified criteria for dimensional analysis and situational analysis.

Chapter 10 – Teaching Grounded Theory

Faculty have a responsibility to prepare the future grounded theorists. This chapter is devoted to teaching grounded theory methods. Teaching approaches that have been published are described. I will also share examples of my own teaching assignments in my qualitative methods courses that I use with my PhD students at the University of Connecticut. For example, in one class assignment, I provide students with some data from one of my grounded theory studies. Using Glaserian methods, they individually start to analyze the data. Time is set aside in class for students to share their analysis.

Chapter 11 – Future of Grounded Theory

Some of the future directions of grounded theory are covered in this final chapter. Perhaps quantitative grounded theory can make more of a presence in the literature. In their book, Glaser and Strauss (1967) put forth the option of also doing quantitative grounded theory. Currently this type of grounded theory lags behind qualitative grounded theory. In 2008 Glaser published an entire book on conducting quantitative grounded theory. Maybe soon grounded theorists will start to conduct more quantitative grounded theory. Mixed method grounded theory studies, which are studies using both qualitative and quantitative data, are beginning to be published. In the future, mixed method grounded theory will become even more popular. Rarely are modifications of a grounded theory seen in literature. It is hoped this will be addressed by more researchers. Use of social media sources for data collection will be another direction for the future.

With the help of Charmaz's constructivist grounded theory, there will be a rise in grounded theory studies that focus on social justice. Positionality and reflexivity are often included in constructivist grounded theory studies. In the future, researchers using other grounded theory approaches are encouraged to incorporate these important concepts in their research. In the future, perhaps some strict lines between grounded theory approaches and epistemological foundations can be loosened. For example, why can't a grounded theorist using a Glaserian approach co-construct the findings of a study with the participants?

References

Beck, C. T. (2023). Teetering on the edge: A third grounded theory modification of postpartum depression. *Advances in Nursing Science*, 46(1), 14–27. https://doi.org/10.1097/ANS.0000000000000432

Bowers, B. J., & Schatzman, L. (2009). Dimensional analysis. In J. M. Morse, P. N. Stern, J. Corbin, B. Bowers, K. Charmaz, & A. E. Clarke (Eds.), *Developing grounded theory: The second generation*. (pp. 86–106). Left Coast Press.

Bowers, B. J., & Schatzman, L. (2021). Dimensional analysis. In J. M. Morse, B. J. Bowers, K. Charmaz, A. E. Clarke, J. Corbin, C. J. Porr, & P. N. Stern (Eds.), *Developing grounded theory: The second generation revisited*. (pp. 111–129). Routledge.

Charmaz, K. (2025). *Constructing grounded theory* (3rd ed.). Sage.

Clarke, A. E., Friese, C., & Washburn, R. S. (2018). *Situational analysis: Grounded theory after the interpretive turn*. Sage.

Glaser, B. G., & Strauss, A. (1967). *The discovery of grounded theory: Strategies for qualitative research*. Aldine de Gruyter.

Morse, J. M., Bowers, B. J., Charmaz, K., Clarke, A. E., Corbin, J., & Porr, C. J. (2021). *Developing grounded theory: The second generation revisited*. Routledge.

Schatzman, L. (1991). Dimensional analysis: Notes on an alternative approach to the grounding of theory in qualitative research. In D. Maines (Ed.), *Social organization and social process: Essays in honor of Anslem Strauss* (pp. 303–314). Aldine de Gruyter.

2

AND SO IT BEGAN

Barney Glaser and Anselm Strauss' Grounded Theory

Dean Helen Nahm of the University of California San Francisco (UCSF) School of Nursing recruited Anselm Strauss (1916–1996), who was a well-known medical sociologist, to strengthen her PhD program in nursing. Strauss had been awarded a grant to study dying patients in California hospitals. Strauss in turn recruited Barney Glaser (1930–2022) to join the faculty at the School of Nursing and work with him on his grant. These two sociologists brought different backgrounds to their collaboration, as can be seen in Table 2.1. Strauss was the senior faculty member and researcher while Glaser was a new PhD. Strauss' graduate education was at the University of Chicago where he was mentored by Herbert Blumer and learned about symbolic interaction. Glaser received his PhD from Columbia University and was mentored by Paul Lazarsfeld and Robert Merton. By combining their quantitative and qualitative expertise, these two sociologists developed grounded theory while working together on the dying in hospitals grant.

Glaser came with a quantitative emphasis. He learned from Lazarsfeld about index formation where Lazersfeld would take questions that focused on the same topic and sum their aggregate values as a group (Glaser, 1998). Next, Lazarsfeld would divide values in thirds or quarters to develop an index with various values like high, medium, and low. Glaser recalled that from the quantitative index formation emerged his constant comparative method for grounded theory where he compared indicators but did not sum them. During his doctoral studies, Glaser also learned about theory construction from Merton and the all-important theoretical coding (Glaser, 1998). After receiving his degree from Stanford University in Sociology, Glaser spent some important time at the University of Paris where he studied literature. He learned explication de texte, a careful reading of text by line-by-line

DOI: 10.4324/9781032695563-2

TABLE 2.1 Background of Glaser and Strauss

	Barney Glaser	*Anselm Strauss*
Life	1930–2022	1916–1996
Education	BS in Sociology (1952) Stanford University Studied contemporary literature & Explication de Text University of Paris University of Freiburg PhD in Sociology (1961) Columbia University	BS in Sociology (1939) University of Virginia Masters in Sociology (1942) University of Chicago PhD in Sociology (1945) University of Chicago
Academic advisors	Lazarsfeld's interchangeability of indices Latent structure analysis/ index formation & constant comparison Merton's theory construction Hans Zetterberg's practical value of social theory and empirical research as basis of theory development	Blumer/symbolic interaction Sociological theory based on real-life solutions Pragmatics
Dissertation	Organizational scientists: Their professional careers	A study of three psychological factors affecting choice of a mate in a college metropolitan population
Paradigm	Quantitative Positivist	Qualitative Symbolic interactionism

comparisons, that helps abstraction, emergence of concepts, and uncovering hidden connections.

Strauss came from a qualitative emphasis at the University of Virginia where he completed his undergraduate degree and learned about Dewey's philosophy of pragmatism. During his doctoral studies at the University of Chicago, Strauss was introduced to the writings of George Herbert Mead and Herbert Blumer, which emphasized symbolic interaction and the significance of interaction for individuals and the symbolic meaning of objects. After graduate school, Strauss discovered again the writings of Dewey on action in response to problematic situations, the importance of the process in events, and relationships of consequences of one action to conditions impacting the next action in a sequence. With his theoretical and philosophical foundation, Strauss might be called a "pragmatist interactionist" (Corbin, 1991, p. 21).

While working together on the dying in hospitals grant and sharing their backgrounds in quantitative and qualitative research, Glaser and Strauss discovered a systematic grounded theory approach to generating substantive theory. At this time in sociology, qualitative research was only viewed as a prelude to quantitative research. Only quantitative research could verify findings and hypotheses. Sociologists underestimated the ability of qualitative research. Glaser and Strauss contended that qualitative research can be used to discover concepts and hypotheses that are related to a substantive area being studied. Qualitative research can help discover a substantive theory that formulated concepts and how they related into hypotheses.

In 1965 Glaser and Strauss' publications began on their new qualitative methodology for developing substantive theory they had initiated in their awareness of dying study (Glaser & Strauss, 1965a). In the appendix to the *Awareness of Dying* book can be found an abbreviated description of their methods of collecting and analyzing data. Two other articles published that year provided a more detailed account. Written by both sociologists was the article, "Discovery of substantive theory: A basic strategy underlying qualitative research" (Glaser & Strauss, 1965b). Glaser (1965) alone published the second article entitled "The constant comparative method of qualitative analysis".

Glaser and Strauss (1967) did not specifically articulate their epistemological perspectives in *The Discovery of Grounded Theory: Strategies for Qualitative Research*. Their use of terms such as verification, a priori, and hypothesis testing implied a traditional positivist approach for their method. Both pragmatism and symbolic interaction, however, underpinned their dying in the hospital's study and helped to develop their grounded theory method. Many held the view that positivism predominated in their method. This was not surprising since in the 1960s grounded theory method assumed the prevailing positivist view of knowledge and quantitative research (Bryant & Charmaz, 2007).

In the first paragraph of their book, Glaser and Strauss stressed that their process of generating theory was independent of the kind of data used. Grounded theory can be developed from both qualitative and quantitative data. In the second half of their book, they focused on generating grounded theory using quantitative data.

Most writing on sociological method has been concerned with how accurate facts can be obtained and how theory can thereby be more rigorously tested. In this book we address ourselves to the equally important enterprise of how the discovery of theory from data, systematically obtained and analyzed in social research, can be furthered. We believe that the discovery of theory from data, which we call grounded theory, is a major task confronting sociology today, for, as we shall try to show, such a theory fits empirical situations, and is understandable to sociologists and laymen alike. Most important, it works and provides us with relevant predictions, explanations, interpretations, and application.

(Glaser & Strauss, 1967, p. 1)

Comparative analysis was the strategic method for generating theory which emphasized theory as a process not a perfected product. The components of theory that comparative analysis generates are first conceptual categories and their properties, followed by hypotheses or general relationships among the categories. Glaser and Strauss defined a category as a conceptual element in a theory, while a property is a conceptual aspect of a category.

Joint collection of data, coding, and analysis are the three operations Glaser and Strauss (1967) stressed that need to be done together. Theoretical sampling is the process for collection of data where the researcher chooses what data to collect next and from whom and this is controlled by the emerging theory. There should be no preconceived theoretical framework guiding this process because it could impede the researcher being theoretically sensitive. Specific to their original grounded theory method is a key aspect regarding where the problem the researcher is investigating must come from. It must emerge from the developing theory. When involved in theoretical sampling, the researcher can control the scope of the developing grounded theory by carefully making choices of types of groups to collect data from. When beginning developing grounded theory, the researcher searches for categories and their properties by minimizing differences in groups being compared but as the theory continues to be generated, maximizing differences among comparative groups are focused on.

Theoretical saturation is the criterion used to judge when to stop sampling from different groups pertinent to a category. Glaser and Strauss (1967, p. 61) defined saturation as when "no additional data are being found whereby the sociologist can develop properties of a category". Once one category is saturated, the researcher moves on to theoretically sampling other groups for another category.

When collecting data, Glaser and Strauss (1967) had specific directions for researchers to follow during interviewing. At first when just beginning generating a grounded theory, interviews consist of open-ended conversations as participants are asked to tell their stories. As the theory develops, the questions become more specific to fill gaps in categories. Interviews should get shorter as the theory develops.

Glaser and Strauss (1967, p. 105) identified four stages in their constant comparative method: "(1) comparing incidents applicable to each category, (2) integrating categories and their properties, (3) delimiting the theory, and (4) writing the theory". In the first stage their defining rule is "while coding an incident for a category, compare it with the previous incidents in the same and different groups coded in the same category" (Glaser & Strauss, 1967, p. 106). Another rule of their constant comparative method is after coding a category a number of times, researchers need to stop coding and write a memo on their ideas. In constant comparative analysis, Glaser and Strauss called for a variety of sources upon which to draw data from: Field research but also documents such as diaries, newspaper accounts, library materials, and observation.

Glaser and Strauss published two more books together before parting ways: *Time for Dying* (1968) and *Status Passage: A Formal Theory* (1971). Glaser left his faculty position at UCSF in the late 1970s and began the Grounded Theory Institute. He offered grounded theory workshops and published multiple books through his publishing company, Sociology Press. Meanwhile Strauss continued on the UCSF faculty until 1987 when he retired and was a professor emeritus until his death in 1996. Glaser died in 2022. Some of Glaser and Strauss' PhD students went on to modify their grounded theory methodology and became known as second-generation grounded theorists. Figure 2.1 shows the bloodline of grounded theory approaches that is the focus of this book.

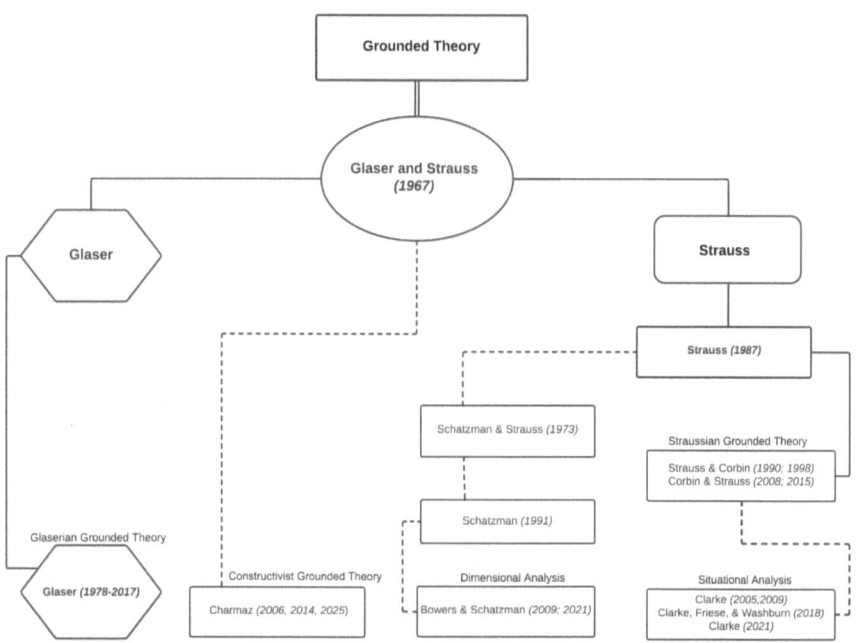

FIGURE 2.1 Grounded Theory's Bloodline

References

Bryant, A., & Charmaz, K. (2007). Grounded theory in historical perspective: An epistemological account. In A. Bryant & K. Charmaz (Eds.), *The SAGE handbook of grounded theory* (pp. 31–57). Sage.

Corbin, J. (1991). Anselm Strauss: An intellectual biography. In D. R. Maines (Ed.), *Social organization and social process: Essays in honor of Anselm Strauss* (pp. 17–42). Aldine de Gruyter.

Glaser, B. G. (1965). The constant comparative method of qualitative analysis. *Social Problems, 12*, 436–445.

Glaser, B. G. (1998). *Doing grounded theory: Issues and discussions.* Sociology Press.

Glaser, B. G., & Strauss, A. (1965a). *Awareness of dying.* Aldine Transaction.

Glaser, B. G., & Strauss, A. (1965b). Discovery of substantive theory: A basic strategy underlying qualitative research. *The American Behavioral Scientist, 8*, 5–12.

Glaser, B. G., & Strauss, A. (1967). *The discovery of grounded theory: Strategies for qualitative research.* Aldine de Gruyter.

Glaser, B. G., & Strauss, A. (1968). *Time for dying.* Aldine Publishing Company.

Glaser, B. G., & Strauss, S. (1971). *Status passage: A formal theory.* Sociology Press.

3

GLASERIAN GROUNDED THEORY

Eleven years after the publication of *The Discovery of Grounded Theory: Strategies for Qualitative Research*, Glaser (1978) on his own published *Theoretical Sensitivity: Advances in the Methodology of Grounded Theory*. He dedicated the book to Strauss. Glaser had two purposes in writing this book. The first was to update the advancements that he had made to the grounded theory methodology since the original publication in 1967 and to take a closer look at theoretical sampling, memoing, substantive and theoretical coding, saturation, and basic social processes. The second purpose was to help develop researchers' theoretical sensitivity which they need to generate substantive grounded theories. Glaser identified that theoretical sensitivity was not focused on in enough depth in *The Discovery of Grounded Theory: Strategies for Qualitative Research*. The beginning step to gain theoretical sensitivity is for the researcher to enter the study with as few predetermined ideas as possible to be sensitive to the data collected without the filter of preexisting hypotheses. To the original criteria for a grounded theory to be fit, relevant, and it must work, Glaser added one more criterion, that being, the theory needs to be readily modifiable from new data.

An element of Glaser's (1978) grounded theory that is controversial with the second-generation grounded theorists is when reviewing the literature should start. Glaser emphasized that reading the literature in the early stages of grounded theory can contaminate researchers' efforts to generate concepts from their data using preconceived concepts. For Glaser, collecting data occurs first. Only when the theory is sufficiently developed, then researchers review the literature and relate the theory to it.

The aim of Glaser's grounded theory is for researchers to explain how the basic social process resolves the discovered basic social psychological problem of the participants in the substantive area being studied. Both inductive

DOI: 10.4324/9781032695563-3

and deductive logic are involved. Grounded theory is inductive as the theory emerges after data are being collected. Deductive logic is also used to identify from the induced codes where to go to next for the comparative group that is needed to be sampled for additional data to develop the theory. Glaser stressed that deductions are not made from preexisting theories in the literature.

With his quantitative background, Glaser viewed data in a positivist fashion where researchers simply observe and analyze it in a straightforward manner (Bryant & Charmaz, 2007). Data emerge. Glaser did not acknowledge the grounded theorist's positionality in the research process.

In *The Discovery of Grounded Theory: Strategies for Qualitative Research*, Glaser and Strauss (1967) included information about coding in general but Glaser (1978) provided more specific details on substantive coding and also added theoretical coding which was not part of Glaser and Strauss' (1967) book. There are two main types of codes that are needed to generate a grounded theory: Substantive and theoretical. In substantive coding, the researcher conceptualizes the empirical data in the area being studied. Substantive coding can be divided into two types: Open and selective. Open coding continues until the researcher identifies a core variable. Then selective coding begins as the researcher limits coding only to those variables related to the core variable. Coding conceptualizes the underlying pattern of empirical indicators in data. Theoretical coding focuses on conceptualizing how the substantive codes relate to each other as hypotheses that are integrated into the grounded theory. In *Theoretical Sensitivity: Advances in the Methodology of Grounded Theory*, Glaser first time presented the 18 coding families to help researchers with theoretical coding (Table 3.1).

TABLE 3.1 Glaser's (1978) 18 Theoretical Coding Families

- The six Cs: Causes, contexts, contingencies, consequences, covariances, and conditions
- Process
- Degree family
- Dimension family
- Type family
- Strategy family
- Interactive family
- Identity-self family
- Cutting point family
- Means-goal family
- Cultural family
- Consensus family
- Mainline family
- Theoretical family
- Ordering or elaboration family
- Unit family
- Reading family
- Models

In *Theoretical Sensitivity: Advances in the Methodology of Grounded Theory*, Glaser expanded discussion of memoing that had not been included in *The Discovery of Grounded Theory: Strategies for Qualitative Research*. Memo writing helps the researcher fill out theoretical properties of the substantive data collected. Memoing helps to define boundaries of a code, the conditions under which it emerged, and the relationship between one property of a code to other properties of the code. Memos also aid in locating the category which is being coded in relationship to other variables. In order to help in sorting memos, Glaser (1978) stressed that each memo needs to be labeled with a title or caption which refers to the category or property that the memo is about. Glaser provided some rules of memoing:

- Keep memos and data separate.
- Always stop coding for writing a memo when the thought occurs.
- Don't be afraid to modify memos as theory develops.
- Keep a list of emergent codes handy.
- If too many memos on different codes appear similar, and if they are the same, collapse the two codes into one code.
- When writing memos discuss conceptually about the substantive codes.
- Indicate "saturation" in memos when the researcher thinks the category is saturated.
- Always be flexible with memoing.

Table 3.2 presents an example of a memo from Laura Foran Lewis' (2014) grounded theory dissertation, "Caregiving for a loved one with dementia". I was her major advisor in her PhD in Nursing Program at the University of Connecticut.

New to Glaser's (1978) expanded and updated grounded theory methodology were details on basic social processes that were not included in the original Glaser and Strauss's (1967) methodology. Researchers generate a grounded theory around a core category which focuses on how the participants resolve the basic problem. Glaser (1978) provided criteria that researchers can use to help identify the core category: (1) it must be central, (2) reoccurs frequently in the data, (3) takes more time to saturate than other categories, (4) relates meaningfully and easily with other categories, (5) has clear implications for a formal theory, (6) has considerable carry through, (7) is completely variable, (8) is a dimension of the problem, (9) prevents two other sources of establishing a core that is not grounded in the data, (10) sees core category in all relations, and (11) can be any kind of theoretical code. Most of the time but not always the core category is a basic social process which is one type of core category. All basic social processes are core variables but not all core variables are basic

TABLE 3.2 Example of a Memo: Caregiving for a Loved One With Dementia

Trying to decipher what the core category is – but I don't think it has emerged just yet. Here are my thoughts so far.

1 The need to be an advocate
   …HAD to be there, mistrust when not there, nurse instead of family, struggle to navigate system

   - Self- advocating
   - Irreplaceable (had to drop everything to be there)
   - Question: Irreplaceable in whose mind? Patients? Caregivers? Health care workers? Other family members?
   - "Vigilant gatekeeper"

2 Role reversal of parent/child relationship – unique to children caring for parents? Challenge of seeing parents as weak/vulnerable/helpless – nothing I could do.

   - Reversing roles
   - Redefining relationships – spouses report no longer sharing "marriage" relationship.

3 Personal sacrifice/strain
   Jobs, marriage, finances, physical health, high stress, reliving same thing over and over, heartbreak … still losing the person you love, can't go anywhere

   - Giving of self
   - All-encompassing
   - Going through the motions
   - Isolation/loneliness

I feel like I may have hit on something with the irreplaceable piece. All others follow this – the caregiver is in a position to accept or reject the all-encompassing role, leading to either distress with acceptance or guilt if unable to become the sole, irreplaceable caregiver. Those who choose this role forewarn others to remember not to be a martyr and to use help, but they are not able themselves to see this when they are caregiving or to do anything about it if they can see it. Dementia and caregiving become their world, and everything else must take a backseat to fill this role to avoid guilt. It is like an unhealthy obsession forced on them. Inescapable until death, when relief finally comes.

Questions for future interviews:

Did you feel like you were the only one who could do this?

Did you ever feel trapped in this role?

Did you feel like others could take your place if you needed a break?

How did this affect our life outside of caregiving?

Source: Lewis (2014, p. 178).

social processes. Phases or stages are the primary properties of basic social processes.

After *Theoretical Sensitivity: Advances in the Methodology of Grounded Theory*, Glaser has gone on to continually publish many books on his grounded theory methodology which he called a set of procedures. In 1998 in *Doing Grounded Theory: Issues and Discussions*, Glaser again emphasized the important aspects of his grounded theory such as when to read the literature. He wrote

> Grounded theory's very strong dicta are a) do not do a literature review in the substantive area and related areas where the research is to be done, and b) when the grounded theory is nearly completed during sorting and writing up, then the literature search in the substantive area can be accomplished and woven into the theory as more data for constant comparison.
>
> *(p. 67)*

Glaser (2013) devoted an entire book to this topic entitled *No Preconceptions: The Grounded Theory Dictum.* Glaser (1998) stressed that his

> Rigor and systematization do not make it an enslaving, forcing methodology ... Grounded theory does not constrain and take over the researcher by forcing strategies and controls. It frees him to run with his or her ongoing discoveries, by constant collecting, coding, and analyzing.
>
> *(pp. 13–14)*

Another reemphasized dictum was to allow the main concern or problem of the participants to emerge.

> It is the first prime organizational feature of the grounded theory research that the researcher is to discover as he enters the field to start his research. Without this problem to begin to organize the research, the researcher will end up with just a list of interesting topics conceptually described but accounting for very little and will not end up with a problem that a theory can account for and that leads to explaining most of the behavior in the area.
>
> *(Glaser, 2013, p. 132)*

The main concern can lead to the core category of the process used to resolve it. Glaser stated that this is the second organizational feature of grounded theory.

Glaser (1998) stressed another of his cardinal rules, "do not tape interviews" (p. 107) especially if researchers are conducting the study on their own without a research team. He went on to explain that the deficits of taping outweigh any benefits. Taping slows data collection and gives too much unnecessary data. Field notes instead of taping were encouraged.

Concentrating on providing researchers with more details about theoretical coding, Glaser (2005) devoted a book to theoretical coding. He widely expanded the 18 families of codes he had listed in 1978. Glaser called for researchers to stay open to emergent theoretical codes beyond the boundaries of their respective disciplines. Examples of possible emergent theoretical codes were amplifying causal looping from economics, bias random walk model from biochemistry, and conjectural causation from political science.

Glaser (2005) stressed that:

> Grounded theory is simply an inductive model for research. It is a paradigm for discovery of what is going on in any particular arena…Whether grounded theory takes on the mantle for the moment of prepositivist, positivist, postpositivist, postmodernism, naturalism, realism etc., will be dependent on its application to the type of data in a specific research.
>
> *(p. 145)*

In 2014 Glaser published *Memoing: A Vital Grounded Theory Procedure* to emphasize its importance from the very start of a grounded theory study. He wrote this book devoted to memoing because "memos are neglected as a grounded theory procedure" (p. 1).

Saturation does not mean the same pattern is seen over and over again in different incidents. For Glaser (2001), saturation is "the conceptualization of comparisons of these incidents which yield different properties of the patterns, until no new properties of the pattern emerge" (p. 191). Saturation is based on the interchangeability of indices. Incidents can be empirically different, but they indicate the same concept and its properties.

In *Emergence vs Forcing: Basics of Grounded Theory Analysis* (1992), Glaser strongly critiqued Strauss and Corbin's (1990) book entitled *Basics of Qualitative Research: Techniques and Procedures for Developing Grounded Theory*. He vehemently asserted their method was not grounded theory but instead resulted in full conceptual description and not a grounded theory. Strauss and Corbin with their axial coding created a coding paradigm of conditions, context, action/interactional strategies, and consequences. Glaser believed that data are forced into this paradigm and are not free to emerge. Glaser's final books were *The Grounded Theory Perspective: Its Origin and Growth* (2016) and *Grounded Descriptions: A No No* (2017). After Strauss' death, Glaser (1991) wrote in honor of Anselm Strauss, "Anselm taught me how to conduct research and analyze data to find out 'what is really going on'. He also taught me that data come first, then theory" (p. 12). In addition to learning how to derive concepts from data from Strauss, Glaser added what he had learned at Columbia University about theoretical coding, theoretical connections, and core categories as critical movers of all other variables in a theory.

Back in 1998, Glaser wrote "in 30 years the definition of grounded theory has not changed. It is still the systematic generation of theory from data" (p. 12). In a panel symposium about grounded theory, Glaser stated that "grounded theory is simply the discovery of emerging patterns in data … All you're doing is looking for patterns of behavior that explain a main concern,

TABLE 3.3 Progression of Glaser's Publication History

Year	Publication
1978	Theoretical Sensitivity: Advances in the Methodology of Grounded Theory
1992	Emergence vs forcing: Basics of Grounded Theory Analysis
1996	Gerund Grounded Theory: The Basic Social Process Dissertation
1998	Doing Grounded Theory: Issues and Discussion
2001	The Grounded Theory Perspective: Conceptualization Contrasted with Description
2003	The Grounded Theory Perspective II: Description's Remodeling of Grounded Theory Methodology
2005	The Grounded Theory Perspective: Theoretical Coding
2007	Doing Formal Grounded Theory: A Proposal
2009	Jargonizing: Using The Grounded Theory Vocabulary
2011	Getting Out of the Data: Grounded Theory Conceptualization
2012	Stop, Write: Writing Grounded Theory
2013	No Preconceptions: The Grounded Theory Dictum
2014	Applying Grounded Theory: A Neglected Option
2014	Memoing: A Vital Grounded Theory Procedure
2016	Grounded Theory Perspective: Its Origin and Growth
2016	The Cry for Help: Preserving Autonomy Doing Grounded Theory for Research
2017	Grounded Descriptions: A No No

and then you name the patterns. Patterns are what people are doing to resolve their main concern" (Walsh et al., 2015, pp. 593–594).

Table 3.3 comprises a list of Glaser's publications.

Modification of Grounded Theory

When a researcher completes a grounded theory study, it does not have complete closure because as new data become available, the theory can be modified. As Glaser (1978; 1998; 2001; 2014) had repeatedly stressed, all grounded theory studies have the potential to be modified. "So the published word is not the final one, but only a pause in the never-ending process of generating theory" (Glaser & Strauss, 1967, p. 40). Grounded theory modification should never stop. Modifiability is one of Glaser's criteria of rigor in a grounded theory study. Basic social processes can be modified based on the changing landscape of the world so as to maintain their continuing relevance. Glaser (2001) clarified that a grounded theory study is not continually modified by testing or being verified, but instead by conceptual generation using new data. In grounded theory the conceptual level leads to modifying the theory as more categories and their properties are developed. The scope of modifying a grounded theory can be increased and controlled by the researcher making conscious choices of groups for comparison (Glaser & Strauss, 1967).

Glaser's famous phrase is "all is data" (1998, p. 8). He explained that whatever is happening in the research landscape and no matter the source, it can be considered as data. As new literature and research findings are published or presented at conferences, these can be used for comparison. Continually comparing the literature as new data are located results in generating new categories and their properties. Modification occurs as these new data from the literature are woven into the grounded theory study. The theory is modified to accommodate the various conditions to increase the grounded theory's completeness and power.

Nathaniel (2021) called for researchers and PhD students to meet the challenge of examining and modifying extant grounded theories based on the changing social and structural processes of today to maintain their relevance when new core problems and processes continue to be identified. Nathaniel and Andrews (2010) asked the question, is Glaser and Strauss' (1965) grounded theory of awareness of dying in need of modification? These researchers compared the original grounded theory to contemporary research results and concluded that it was not in need of modification. Its relevance still remained.

My Example of Classic Grounded Theory

I conducted "Releasing the pause button: Mothering twins during the first year of life" (Beck, 2002, p. 596) to answer the following two research questions:

1 What is the specific social psychological problem mothers of twins encounter during the first year after birth?
2 What social psychological process do mothers of twins use to resolve this fundamental problem?

I used Glaserian grounded theory approach with purposive and theoretical sampling to obtain my 13 participants. Unstructured interviews and participant observation were the two data sources. I did participant observation in a Parents of Multiples Support Group. I conducted 13 private interviews in participants' homes where I stayed after the interviews were completed for participant observation there e.g., helping to feed the twins. An example illustrating the use of theoretical sampling focused on what mothers termed "the blur period". When I first started interviewing, I purposely chose mothers whose twins were close to 1-year-old, so they would have the past year to reflect on their experiences. Participants spoke of the "blur period" during the first few months after giving birth. When I asked them to please tell me more about this experience, they could not because "it was such a blur". Theoretical sampling next directed me to interviewing mothers who were in this blur period to find out more about it. I then recruited mothers of twins who were in the first 2-3 months after giving birth. My interviewing process continually

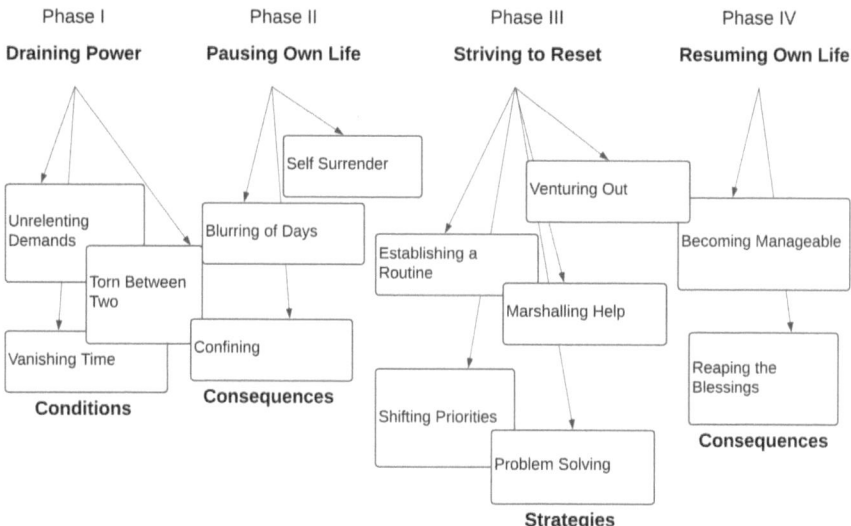

FIGURE 3.1   Four Phases of Releasing the Pause Button

Source: Reprinted with permission from Beck (2002, p. 599).

changed as the grounded theory developed. First, I began the interviews with general questions like, can you please tell me what it is like being a mother of twins? As the core category was discovered, my questions guiding my interviews became more specific to help fill in the categories and their properties.

The basic problem I discovered of mothering twins during the first year after giving birth was Life on Hold. Releasing the pause button was the basic social psychological process of mothering twins over the first 12 months of life. This process entailed four phases (Figure 3.1) as mothers progressed through resuming their lives. These four phases included: (1) Draining Power, (2) Pausing Own Life, (3) Striving to Reset, and (4) Resuming Own Life. Draining Power was the first phase where women's physical and emotional endurance were taxed to the limit. It consisted of three categories: Unrelenting Demands, Vanishing Time, and Torn between Two Infants. Phase 2, Pausing Own Life, consisted of three categories which were the consequences of the conditions in Phase 1. These three categories were Burring of Days, Confining, and Self-Surrender. In Phase 3, Striving to Reset, mothers used five strategies to help resolve their basic problem: Establishing a Routine, Shifting Priorities, Marshaling Help, Problem Solving, and Venturing Out. The consequences in Phase 2 were conditions that led to strategies the mothers used. Conditions, consequences, and strategies were theoretical codes used in this grounded theory to connect the categories. The final Phase 4 of Releasing the Pause Button was Resuming Own Life that consisted of two consequences of the strategies used in Phase 3: Becoming Manageable and Reaping the Blessings.

This four-phase process women used to resume their lives caring for twins over the first 12 months of the infants' lives can be used by healthcare professionals to locate where in the process mothers of multiples are. Specific interventions can then be designed and implemented to target different phases of this substantive theory. In this grounded theory, the theoretical code of a cutting point was identified. The cutting point was 3 months postpartum when life began to be a bit more manageable caring for twins as they began to start to sleep through the night.

My Example of Grounded Theory Modification

In 1993 I conducted my original grounded theory study of postpartum depression called, Teetering on the Edge (Beck, 1993). The sample consisted of women who were all married, White, and had attended a local postpartum depression support group. The version of grounded theory I used was classic grounded theory (Glaser, 1978; Glaser & Strauss, 1967). Data collection involved not only in-depth interviews but also participant observation for 18 months in the postpartum depression support group. Loss of control was the basic social psychological problem in postpartum depression. Mothers had absolutely no control over their emotions, thought processes, or actions. The basic social psychological process women used to resolve this basic problem I entitled, Teetering on the Edge, which made reference to their walking a fine line between sanity and insanity each day. This involved a four-stage process: (1) Encountering Terror, (2) Dying of Self, (3) Struggling to Survive, and (4) Regaining Control (Figure 3.2). This original grounded theory study had limited transferability since the participants were all White women living in the United States.

Almost 15 years later, I conducted the first modification of Teetering on the Edge (Beck, 2007) to increase the scope of the theory to include women living in other countries and from different cultures. Since 1993, ten qualitative studies of women's experiences of postpartum depression in other countries/ethnicities had been published. The findings of these ten qualitative studies were used as new data to modify my grounded theory study. In this first modification, the categories under each of the four stages remained the same. Now under each phase, I listed the countries outside the United States where the new data had been conducted and the mothers had endorsed the categories.

Five years later, I conducted a second grounded theory modification of Teetering on the Edge to now include 17 more transcultural qualitative studies of women's experiences of postpartum depression that had been published since my first modification (Beck, 2012). In this second modification, the same four stages remained. The one modification was made to the first stage, Encountering Terror, where I added two new categories: Emotional Lability and Somatic

The Four Stage Process of Teetering on the Edge

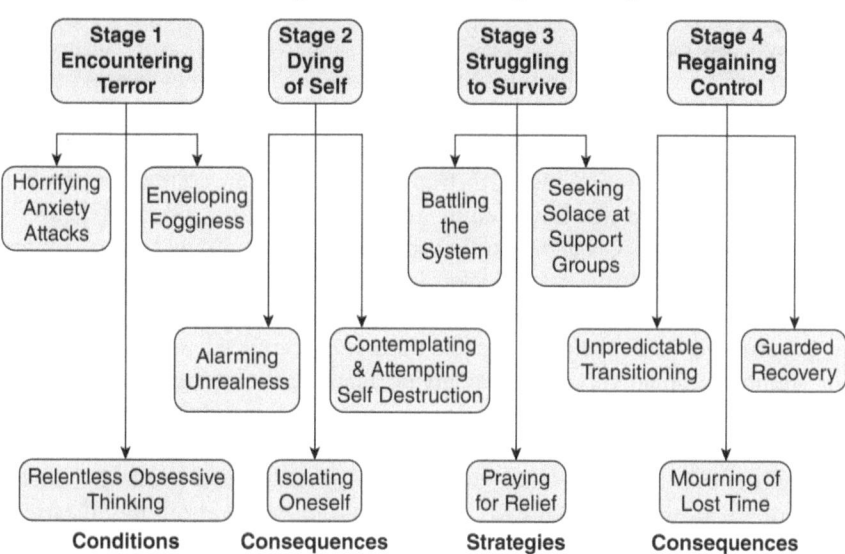

FIGURE 3.2   Four Stage Process of Teetering on the Edge

Source: From Beck, C.T. (1993), Teetering on the Edge: A Substantive Theory of Postpartum Depression. Nursing Research.

Expressions. In the original grounded theory study, mood swings and changes in emotions that women could not control had been addressed under the basic problem of loss of control. These data from the new 17 qualitative studies led to making a separate category to focus more attention on emotional lability. The other category added to Stage 1 was a new category called Somatic Expressions. Women from countries such as Taiwan, Indonesia, India, Democratic Republic of Congo, and Bangladesh often used somatic terms to describe their experiences of postpartum depression. This second modification continued to increase Teetering on the Edge's completeness and power.

A decade later, I tackled the third modification of my grounded theory. This time I set my sights on increasing the completeness of Teetering on the Edge to include data from 13 qualitative studies that specifically focused on immigrant and refugee women's experiences of postpartum depression (Beck, 2023). Participants in these studies were living in the following countries: Canada, United Kingdom, Australia, and on the Thai Myanmar border. The four stages of Teetering on the Edge remained unchanged. With the addition of these new data from the 13 qualitative studies, modifications to Stage 3, Struggling to Survive, were made. Two new categories were added to increase the scope of the grounded theory to include immigrant and refugee women's postpartum depression experiences.

In Stage 3, Struggling to Survive, was where most of the data shared by immigrant and refugee mothers' postpartum depression experiences focused. The two new categories added to Stage 3 were Battling Self and Culture, and Barriers to Sources of Support. Mothers explained that they battled within themselves whether or not to disclose they were experiencing postpartum depression and to ask for help. Cultural stigma attached to discussing mental health issues after giving birth was a barrier in their cultures for seeking the help women needed from family and mental health professionals. In the second new category, Barriers to Sources of Support, immigrant and refugee mothers faced multiple roadblocks. Language was a barrier that hindered mothers from much needed support from healthcare professionals. Also, being separated from their families in their home country impacted the lack of support women received after giving birth. Lack of support from their partners during their postpartum depression compounded an already difficult situation. Some women reported verbal and physical abuse.

Figures 3.3–3.6 show each of the four stages of this grounded theory illustrating how each stage was adjusted based on all three modifications. Under each category in each stage are listed the host countries where women shared experiencing that category.

Modifications of a grounded theory can be viewed as using a kaleidoscope (Beck, 2023). As researchers and clinicians turn the kaleidoscope, new patterns are created. The original pattern viewed women's postpartum depression experiences that concentrated on White, non-Hispanic women in the

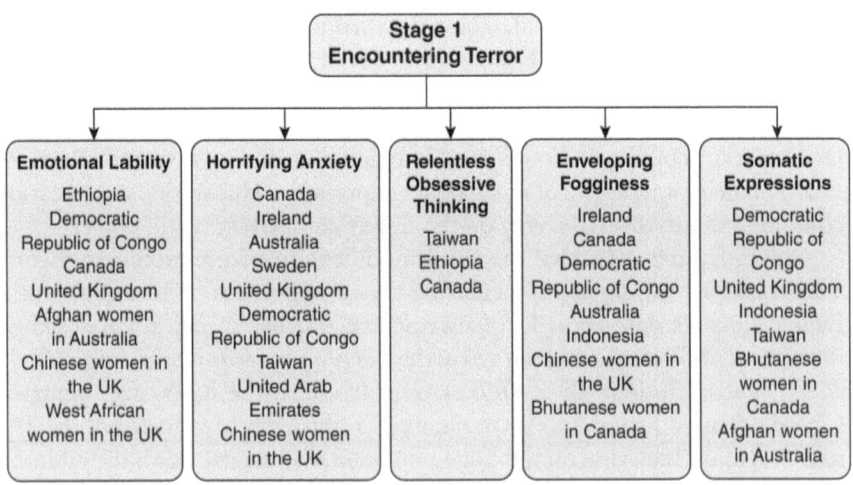

FIGURE 3.3 Third modification of Teetering on the Edge: Stage 1

Source: Beck, C.T. (2023), Teetering on the Edge: A Third Grounded Theory Modification of Postpartum Depression. Advances in Nursing Science.

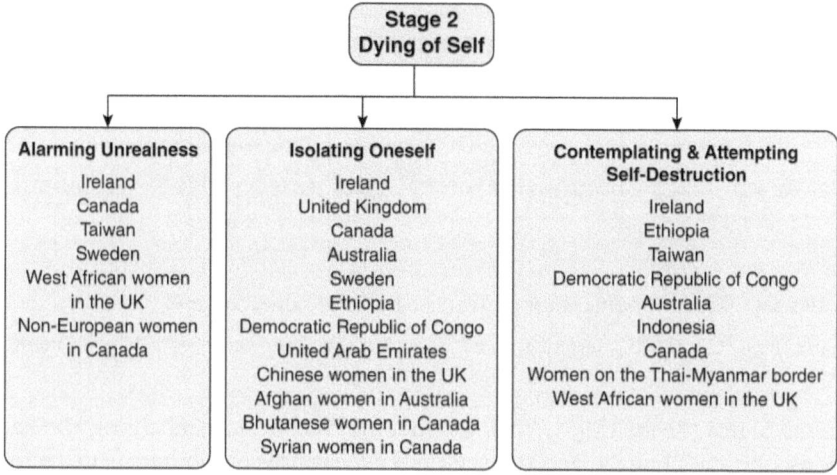

FIGURE 3.4 Third modification of Teetering on the Edge: Stage 2

Source: Beck, C.T. (2023), Teetering on the Edge: A Third Grounded Theory Modification of Postpartum Depression. Advances in Nursing Science.

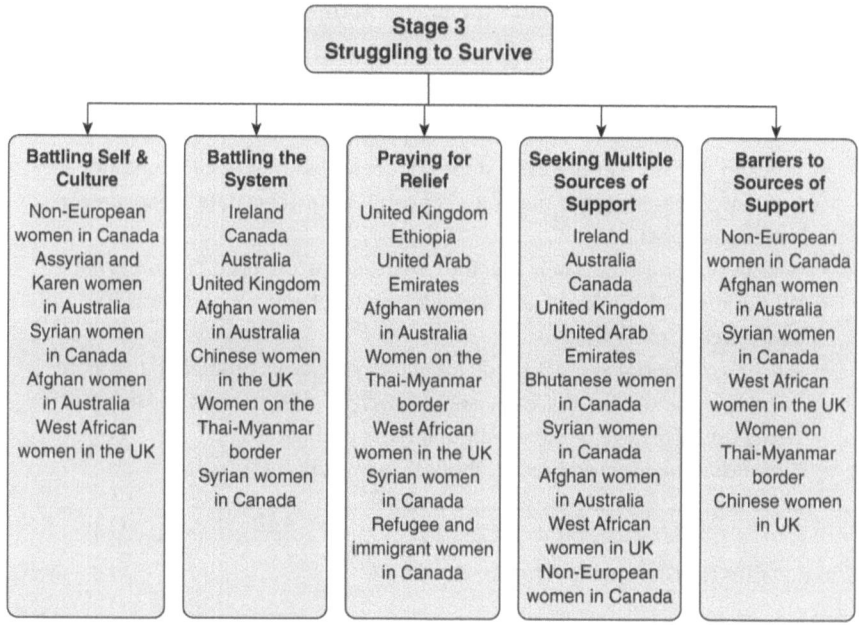

FIGURE 3.5 Third modification of Teetering on the Edge: Stage 3

Source: Beck, C.T. (2023), Teetering on the Edge: A Third Grounded Theory Modification of Postpartum Depression. Advances in Nursing Science.

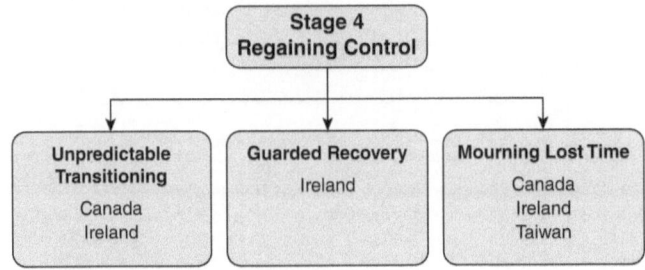

FIGURE 3.6 Third modification of Teetering on the Edge: Stage 4

Source: Beck, C.T. (2023), Teetering on the Edge: A Third Grounded Theory Modification of Postpartum Depression. Advances in Nursing Science.

United States (Beck, 1993). With the first and second modifications, the kaleidoscope lens changed and transcultural experiences of mothers from countries outside the United States came into focus. Rotating the kaleidoscope lens for the third modification brought into focus a different pattern, this time specifically for immigrant and refugee mothers' postpartum depression experiences. The scope and complexity of Teetering on the Edge have been expanded. With these three modifications, specific interventions to help mothers experiencing postpartum depression can be developed depending on which lens of the kaleidoscope clinicians look through.

KEY POINTS IN GLASERIAN GROUNDED THEORY

- Reading literature in the early stages of grounded theory can contaminate a researcher's efforts to generate concepts from their data using preconceived concepts.
- Selective coding begins only after the researcher has identified the core variable.
- All basic social processes are core variables but not all core variables are basic social processes.
- Glaser's methodology focuses on identifying the basic problem participants experience and then the basic social psychological process those participants use to resolve or cope with that basic problem.
- Grounded theory modification should never stop.

Current Classic Grounded Theory Books

Holton and Walsh have published two books on classic grounded theory (Holton & Walsh, 2017; Walsh et al., 2020). Holton attended many of Glaser's troubleshooting seminars in addition to offering some seminars herself internationally. Holton is a past editor-in-chief of *The Grounded Theory Review*.

Glaser had suggested that Holton write a "troubleshooting book based on the many questions and blocks to doing classic grounded theory that the novice researcher encounters" (Holton & Walsh, 2017, p. xvii). At the end of the preface of their book, Walsh wrote "the present book aims to give a clear and savory taste of classic grounded theory and its fundamentals. Ultimately, it should motivate readers to start reading, or to read again with fresh eyes, Barney Glaser's seminal publications" (p. xix). Holton (2007) supported Glaser's view that his classic grounded theory methodology is epistemologically and ontologically neutral. Grounded theory can be used by researchers irrespective of their philosophical positioning (Holton & Walsh, 2017). Holton and Walsh identified as critical realists. In the second book, Walsh et al. (2020) focused on how to conduct classic grounded theory for business and management students. Classic grounded theory permits the creativity of researchers' some freedom while providing them with essential guidelines. Walsh, Holton, and Mourmant are all professors in Schools of Management in Canada and France. Urquhart (2023) published the second edition of her classic grounded theory book, *Grounded Theory for Qualitative Research*. Her discipline is also Business.

In 2022 Simmons published his book, *Experiencing Grounded Theory: A Comprehensive Guide to Learning, Doing, Mentoring, Teaching, and Applying Grounded Theory*, which focused on his experiences conducting, teaching, and mentoring classic grounded theory. He was a PhD student of both Glaser and Strauss at University of California San Francisco (UCSF). He had a strong preference for Glaser's classic grounded theory and has been teaching classic grounded theory for decades.

There is one journal that is dedicated to advancing classic grounded theory and scholarship. It is *The Grounded Theory Review* which is published by the Institute for Research and Theory Methodologies (RTM). The journal is housed within the Glaser Center for Grounded Theory at RTM. The purpose of this center is to support and educate students, faculty, and researchers worldwide to learn Glaserian grounded theory.

Interdisciplinary Examples of Classic Grounded Theory

From the discipline of Social Work, Sun (2022, p. 50) conducted a classic grounded theory study of Filipino factory workers in Taiwan. Specifically, his study addressed the following two research questions:

1 What main concern emerges from Filipino factory workers' migration experiences?
2 How do Filipino factory workers continually resolve this main concern?

Using substantive and theoretical coding and memo writing, the main concern of Filipino factory works discovered was inequality which included a collection of problems and hardships. All the participants shared some form of discrimination and those who worked in smaller family-owned factories reported more abuse than those who worked in larger corporate-owned factories. Working conditions consisted of long hours and verbally abusive employers. Despite Filipino workers having longer hours than Taiwanese workers, migrant workers received lower salaries and fewer benefits. Harsh brokers, who were private intermediaries hired by employers to manage the workers' lives, were another source of inequality. Transcending inequality was the pattern of behavior that Filipino factory workers used to continually resolve their main concern of inequality. Transcending inequality consisted of three overlapping dimensions: Coping, bonding, and serving. Two strategies were involved in coping: Reframing and questioning. Bonding, the second dimension involved forming social relations. Serving, in the context of religious involvement, was the third dimension of transcending inequality. "Serving towards people or God is motivated by opportunities to be thankful, to receive, and to give, which lead to personal and spiritual meaning" (p. 56).

From the discipline of Business, Haslam's (2023) classic grounded theory study in marketing took place in the United Kingdom. He collected data in a high-profile but small management consulting firm where he spent 2 months working on site. This was followed by a period of 9 months where he made additional visits to gather more data from interviews with six staff members of the firm to help investigate marketing behavior of management consultants. Haslam discovered the core variable of personal legitimizing which was a basic social process by which individuals manipulated situations to meet their own agendas. This process consisted of two groups of behaviors: obstructing existing marketing activity and driving new marketing activity. Each of these groups of behaviors had three categories within them. In obstructing existing marketing activity, the manager moved to prevent marketing ideas from being adopted. This consisted of the following three categories: Stigmatizing, pseudo endorsing, and smokescreening. The second behavior group of driving new marketing activity included the categories of latching on, self-indulging, and bragging. In describing his grounded theory, Haslam included detailed memoing to help illustrate his data analysis process using Glaserian grounded theory.

Didier et al. (2024a), from Health Sciences, conducted a Glaserian grounded theory study entitled "protecting personhood in two adult surgery departments in Switzerland". Data collection included individual face-to-face interviews with 32 patients regarding their interactions and relationships with interprofessional healthcare teams. Patients' main concern was to continually ensure they protected their own personhood so they received optimal care. The basic social process of protecting personhood consisted of four stages: Introspection, preservation, rupture, and reconciliation. During introspection, hospitalized patients become aware of themselves as persons and patients. During the stage of preservation, patients find a balance between their sense of personhood and patienthood. Rupture occurs when patients experience an imbalance between their sense of personhood and patienthood. In the fourth stage of reconciliation, their personhood is restored.

In *Theoretical Sensitivity: Advances in the Methodology of Grounded Theory*, Glaser (1978) offered the option of constructing typologies as part of his grounded theory analysis. Typologies are not often reported in published studies using classic grounded theory studies. In further analyzing their data, Didier et al. (2024b) identified a typology of specific types of behaviors of patients in response to clinicians' attitudes and behaviors toward patient expectations. Three distinct types of patients' anticipatory behaviors in their quest to receive optimal care were identified: Propitiation, vigilance, and confidence. Different types of patients were distinguished based on their position on the continuum of control, their level of trust with clinicians, and their prior experiences. Propitiation referred to appeasing healthcare providers or making them happy by acting a certain way. Vigilant behavior occurred in some patients who anticipated some apprehension with care moments. This apprehension could come from the patient's personality that was controlling and vigilant by nature, anxiety regarding hospitalization, or anxious by nature. Confidence was the third specific type of behavior in Didier et al.'s typology. The patients who displayed confident behaviors had experienced positive care from clinicians recently or in the past.

From the Nursing discipline, Wood (2025) conducted a Glaserian grounded theory of the transition to survivorship in older adult blood cancer survivors. She recruited 17 participants from the United States and Canada from the Leukemia and Lymphoma Society Community. Participants participated in in-depth interviews via zoom. Wood used substantive and theoretical coding, memoing, and theoretical sampling. The main concern Wood discovered of older adult blood cancer survivors was losing their sense of self. The core category that emerged was reclaiming self-balancing on a tightrope across time. This basic social process consisted of a six-phase transition to survivorship: Receiving a blood cancer diagnosis, finding bearings, reclaiming self, persevering through, realizing a transition, and living in a new reality.

End-of-Chapter Student Exercise

Skim the table of contents of the studies published in *The Grounded Theory Review* for the past 5 years. Select one study of interest to you and comment on its methodology using the following questions as a guide:

1 Did the researchers follow Glaser's grounded theory methodology? If not, which aspects of his methodology were not followed?
2 What was the research question(s)? Was it congruent with Glaser's grounded theory approach?

3 Was the sampling technique appropriate for Glaser's grounded theory approach?
4 Was the data collection technique appropriate for Glaser's grounded theory approach?
5 Did the researchers adequately describe the process used to analyze their data? Was it appropriate for Glaser's grounded theory approach?
6 Did the researchers report discovering the basic problem? If so, what was it?
7 Did the researchers discover the core variable? Was it a basic social process?
8 If you were to conduct this grounded theory study using Glaser's approach, are there any aspects of it you would change to strengthen its methodology?

References

Beck, C. T. (1993). Teetering on the edge: A substantive theory of postpartum depression. *Nursing Research*, 42, 42–48.

Beck, C. T. (2002). Releasing the pause button: Mothering twins during the first year of life. *Qualitative Health Research*, 12, 593–608. https://doi.org/10.1177/104973202129120124

Beck, C. T. (2007). Exemplar: Teetering on the edge: A continually emerging theory of postpartum depression. In P. L. Munhall (Ed.), *Nursing research: A qualitative perspective* (pp. 273–292). Jones & Bartlett.

Beck, C. T. (2012). Exemplar: Teetering on the edge: A second grounded theory modification (p.257–284). In P.L. Munhall (Ed.), *Nursing research: A qualitative perspective* (5th ed.). Jones & Bartlett Publishers.

Beck, C. T. (2023). Teetering on the edge: A third grounded theory modification of postpartum depression. *Advances in Nursing Science*, 46(1), 14–27. https://doi.org/10.1097/ANS.0000000000000432

Bryant, A., & Charmaz, K. (2007). Grounded theory in historical perspective: An epistemological account. In A. Bryant & K. Charmaz (Eds.), *The SAGE handbook of grounded theory* (pp. 31–57). Sage.

Didier, A., Nathaniel, A., Scott, H., Look, S., Benaroyo, L., & Zumstein-Shaha, M. (2024a). Protecting personhood: A classic grounded theory. *Grounded Theory Review*, 23(1), 36–70.

Didier, A., Nathaniel, A., Scott, H., & Zumstein-Shaha, M. (2024b). Patient behaviors: A grounded theory typology. *Grounded Theory Review*, 23(2), 6–29.

Glaser, B. G. (1978). *Theoretical sensitivity: Advances in the methodology of grounded theory*. Sociology Press.

Glaser, B. G. (1991). Honor of Anselm Strauss: Collaboration. In D. R. Maines (Ed.), *Social organization and social process: Essays in honor of Anselm Strauss* (pp.11–16). De Gruyter.

Glaser, B. G. (1992). *Emergence vs forcing: Basics of grounded theory analysis*. Sociology Press.

Glaser, B. G. (1998). *Doing grounded theory: Issues and discussions*. Sociology Press.

Glaser, B. G. (2001). *The grounded theory perspective: Conceptualization contrasted with description*. Sociology Press.

Glaser, B. G. (2005). *The grounded theory perspective III: Theoretical coding*. Sociology Press.

Glaser, B. G. (2013). *No preconceptions: The grounded theory dictum*. Sociology Press.

Glaser, B. G. (2014). *Memoing: A vital grounded theory procedure*. Sociology Press.

Glaser, B. G. (2016). *The grounded theory perspective: Its origin and growth*. Sociology Press.

Glaser, B. G. (2017). *Grounded descriptions: A no no*. Sociology Press.

Glaser, B. G., & Strauss, A. (1965). *Awareness of dying*. Aldine Transaction.

Glaser, B. G., & Strauss, A. (1967). *The discovery of grounded theory: Strategies for qualitative research*. Aldine de Gruyter.

Haslam, S. (2023). Personal legitimizing: A perspective of marketing management. *Grounded Theory Review*, 22(2), 25–44.

Holton, J. A. (2007). The coding process and its challenges. In A. Bryant & K. Charmaz (Eds.), *The Sage handbook of grounded theory* (pp. 265–289). Sage.

Holton, J. A., & Walsh, I. (2017). *Classic grounded theory: Applications with qualitative & quantitative data*. Sage.

Lewis, L. F. (2014). *Caregiving for a loved one with dementia at the end of life: An emergent theory of the basic social psychological process of rediscovering*. Unpublished Dissertation University of Connecticut.

Nathaniel, A. (2021). The value of modifiability. *The Grounded Theory Review*, 20(2), 1–3.

Nathaniel, A. K., & Andrews, T. (2010). The modifiability of grounded theory. *The Grounded Theory Review*, 9(1), 65–77.

Simmons, O. E. (2022). *Experiencing grounded theory: A comprehensive guide to learning, doing, mentoring, teaching, and applying grounded theory*. Brown Walker Press.

Strauss, A., & Corbin, J. (1990). *Basics of qualitative research: Grounded theory procedures and techniques*. Sage.

Sun, C. P. (2022). Transcending inequality: A classic ground theory of Filipino factory workers in Taiwan. *The Grounded Theory Review*, 21(2), 49–68.

Urquhart, C. (2023). *Grounded theory for qualitative research*. Sage.

Walsh, I., Holton, J. A., Bailyn, L., Fernandez, W., Levina, N., & Glaser, B. (2015). What grounded theory is…A critically reflective conversation among scholars. *Organizational Research Methods*, 18(4), 581–599. https://doi.org/10.1177/1094428114565028

Walsh, I., Holton, J. A., & Mourmant, G. (2020). *Conducting classic grounded theory for business and management students*. Sage.

Wood, S. K. (2025). Reclaiming self-balancing on a tightrope across time: A grounded theory of transition to survivorship in older adult blood cancer survivors. *Journal of Advanced Nursing*, 81, 366–382. https://doi.org/10.1111/jan.16200

4

STRAUSSIAN GROUNDED THEORY

Strauss' first book after parting ways with Glaser was written with Schatzman and was entitled *Field Research: Strategies for a Natural Sociology* (Schatzman & Strauss, 1973). Next in Strauss' (1987) book, *Qualitative Analysis for Social Scientists*, he first introduced his paradigm where he integrated process and structural conditions and placed action in structural context. This was the first book on grounded theory that Strauss wrote since the publication of his book *The Discovery of Grounded Theory: Strategies for Qualitative Research* with Glaser in 1967. In the preface of his qualitative analysis book, Strauss (1987, p. xiv) wrote that there were some differences between his and Glaser's "actual carrying out of research, but the differences are minor". Glaser would disagree with that statement. Strauss went on to explain that he was very much indebted to Glaser for his continued evolution of grounded theory. Also in the preface of his book, Strauss explained that, with permission, the second half of his first chapter was essentially from Glaser's *Theoretical Sensitivity: Advances in the Methodology of Grounded Theory* (1978) "except for some amplifications" (p. xiv). Some of these "amplifications" involved concentrating on a coding paradigm of conditions, interactions, strategies, and consequences and adding a new type of coding – axial coding. This coding revolves around a researcher's analysis around the axis of one category at a time. Strauss labeled axial coding as an essential aspect of open coding. Both the coding paradigm and axial coding made their way into Strauss' first edition of his grounded theory book with Corbin.

For Strauss grounded theory "is not really a specific method or technique, Rather, it is a style of doing qualitative analysis that includes a number of distinct features, such as theoretical sampling, and certain methodological guidelines, such as the making of constant comparisons and the use of a

DOI: 10.4324/9781032695563-4

coding paradigm, to ensure conceptual development and density" (Strauss, 1987, p. 5). According to Strauss, grounded theory analysis involves three processes of induction, deduction, and verification. In induction the researchers' actions lead to discovering a hypothesis. Researchers have a hunch or idea and they develop a hypothesis and then assess whether it works or not, for instance, for a type of relationship or strategy. Deduction refers to the researchers' drawing implications from their hypotheses for verification. In verification, the researchers find out if the hypothesis is totally or partially supported or not at all. For theory development, Strauss stressed that all three processes are essential. It was not until the second generation of grounded theorists that abduction was added to the grounded theory methodology.

In the first edition of *Basics of Qualitative Research: Techniques and Procedures for Developing Grounded Theory* (1990), Strauss teamed up with Juliet Corbin, a nurse, who had completed a post doctorate in the Department of Social and Behavioral Sciences at University of California San Francisco (UCSF) under the direction of Strauss. In the preface, they stated that there were some further differences in terminology and procedures from Glaser's (1978) *Theoretical Sensitivity: Advances in the Methodology of Grounded Theory* and Strauss's (1987) *Qualitative Analysis for Social Scientists* book. Strauss and Corbin (1990) explained that the procedure and techniques were now spelled out step-by-step in greater detail to help researchers learn their qualitative analysis.

For Strauss and Corbin, there are several sources of research problems: Suggested or assigned research problems, personal and professional experience, and technical literature. Unlike Glaser (1978), the basic problem is not discovered during the process of analyzing the data. Their research question also differs from Glaser's (1978) research questions. For Glaser, the questions that are asked are (1) what is the central concern or basic problem and (2) what is the process used to resolve the problem. For Strauss and Corbin, in a grounded theory study, the research question "is a statement that identifies the phenomenon to be studied" (1990, p. 38). The research question starts as an open and broad one to allow flexibility in investigating the phenomenon in depth. The research question can become more focused as the study progresses.

Strauss and Corbin's (1990) use of the literature also differs from Glaser's (1978) view. Unlike Glaser, Strauss and Corbin explained that researchers will come to the start of their study with some background from technical literature like prior research reports. It is important to use this literature but there is no need to review all the literature beforehand. Strauss and Corbin described that "we do not want to be so steeped in the literature as to be constrained and even stifled in terms of creative efforts by our knowledge of it!" (p. 50). They offered some uses of technical literature in grounded theory research. It can stimulate theoretical sensitivity, questions, provide approaches for interpreting data, direct theoretical sampling, be used as secondary sources of data, and supplementary validation.

Strauss and Corbin's (1990) analysis involved three types of coding: Open, axial, and selective. Their first step in analysis focuses on open coding which involves breaking down, comparing and categorizing data, and conceptualizing the data. As researchers develop a category, they look for its properties or characteristics. Each property is dimensionalized along a continuum. Open coding can be accomplished in several ways: Line-by-line analysis, sentence or paragraph, and the entire document. Axial coding involves putting the data back together. Connections are made between categories. Strauss and Corbin (1990) accomplish axial coding by means of using their coding paradigm of conditions, context, action/interactional strategies, and consequences. This paradigm model aids researchers in linking subcategories to a category in a set of relationships and in relating categories to the core category.

Strauss and Corbin (1990) define selective coding as:

The process of selecting the core category, systematically relating it to other categories, validating those relationships, and filling in categories that need further refinement and development.

(p. 116)

Their selective coding differs from Glaser's selective coding which only begins after a core category is selected.

Process involves researchers linking the action/interactional sequences in their developing grounded theory as they evolve overtime. Stages or phrases are one way that process can be conceptualized. Theoretical sampling in the first edition of *Basics of Qualitative Research: Techniques and Procedures for Developing Grounded Theory* was divided into sampling in open coding, axial coding, and selective coding. Strauss and Corbin (1990) called sampling in selective coding, discriminate sampling, when researchers choose participants, sites, and documents that will help verify the story line, identify relationships among categories, and fill data in thinly developed categories.

Important elements of analysis besides the constant comparative method are memoing and diagramming which help move the developing grounded theory from description to conceptualization. Strauss and Corbin (1990) represented their conditional matrix as a set of circles with each one inside the other circle. Their matrix is a tool for sensitizing researchers to the range of conditions and consequences that can be in the context. Each level corresponds to various aspects of the world. Starting with the outermost circle and going inward the levels included: International, national, community, organizational and institutional level, sub-organizational and sub-institutional, group, individual, and collective, interaction and in the center of the circle is action pertaining to a phenomenon. Strauss and Corbin stressed that no matter what the level of a phenomenon is located at, that phenomenon is in a conditional relationship to the different levels above and below it.

Before publishing the second edition of *Basics of Qualitative Research: Techniques and Procedures for Developing Grounded Theory*, Strauss (1993) published *Continual Permutations of Action*. In the introduction, he shared a biography of himself and his slow recognition of the significance of pragmatism's action scheme on his thinking.

> I began to comprehend the links among complexity, action/interaction, and the research methodology we [he and Glaser] had fathered. It did not take very much, thereafter, for Fritz Schuetze and Hans- Georg Soeffner, and later Juliet Corbin, to convince me that a theory of action might lie at the heart of my sociology.
>
> *(p. 12)*

Strauss realized that it was "clear that a list of assumptions about action and interaction obviously derived from pragmatism have run like a red thread through my research" (1993, p. 335). Table 4.1 consists of a list of key assumptions that provide the foundation of Strauss' grounded theory approach and conditional matrix (Strauss, 1993, pp. 23–44). He explained that his conditional matrix analysis was essential for conducting research with an interactionist theory of action. "A conditional matrix and its corresponding diagram are ways of conceptualizing, discovering, and keeping track of the conditions that bear on whatever phenomenon-as defined by the researcher-and its associated interactions that are under study" (Strauss, 1993, p. 60). He went on to say that "this burden lies squarely on the researcher's shoulders, but the concepts of conditional matrix and conditional paths should be helpful" (p. 65).

Strauss (1993) also elaborated on the importance of social worlds and arenas. As you will read in a later chapter, Clarke et al.'s (2018) situational analysis builds on Strauss' social worlds and arenas. Instead of focusing on social structures like most sociologists at that time did, Strauss called for viewing the concept of social worlds as one of the major features of contemporary society to help understand the complexities in collective actions. Social worlds often have subworlds and their relationship to each other needs to be a focus. These social world processes that are linked together lead to complexity. Strauss explained that the concept of arena refers to "the interaction by social worlds around issues where actions concerning these are being debated, fought over, negotiated, manipulated, and even coerced within and among the social worlds" (p. 226).

The second edition of *Basics of Qualitative Research: Techniques and Procedures for Developing Grounded Theory* (Strauss & Corbin, 1998) was

TABLE 4.1 Strauss' List of 19 Assumptions of Interactionist Theory

1   No action is possible without a body.

2   Actions are embedded in interactions – past, present, and imagined future. Thus, actions also carry meanings and are locatable within systems of meanings. Actions may generate further meanings, both with regard to further actions and the interactions in which they are embedded.

3   During early childhood and continuing all through life, humans develop selves that enter into virtually all their actions and in a variety of ways.

4   Meanings (symbols) are aspects of interaction and are related to others within systems of meanings (symbols). Interactions generate new meanings and symbols as well as alter and maintain old ones.

5   The external world is a symbolic representation, a "symbolic universe". Both this and the interior worlds are created and re-created through interaction. In effect there is no divide between external and interior world.

6   Actions (overt and covert) may be preceded, accompanied, and/or succeeded by reflexive interactions. These actions may be one's own or those of other actors. Especially important is that in many actions the future is included in the action.

7   Actions are not necessarily rational: Many are nonrational or, in common parlance, "irrational". Yet rational action may be mistakenly perceived as not so by other actors.

8   Action has emotional aspects: To conceive of emotion as distinguishable from action, as entitles accompanying action, is to reify those aspects of action.

9   Actions are characterized by temporality, for they constitute courses of action of varying duration. Various actors' interpretations of the temporal aspects of an action may differ, according to other actors' respective perspectives; these interpretations may also change as the action proceeds.

10   Courses of interaction are definable into sequences, sometimes classified into stages or phases. Definitions arise out of identical or shared perspectives or must be negotiated.

11   Means-ends analytic schemes are usually not appropriate for understanding action and interaction.

12   Contingencies are likely to arise during a course of action. These can bring about change in its duration, pace, and even intent, which may alter the structure and process of interaction.

13   Interactions may be followed by reviewals of actions, one's own and those of others, as well as projections of future ones. The reviewals and evaluations made along the interactional course may affect a partial or even complete recasting of it.

14   The embeddedness in interaction of an action implies an intersection of actions. The interaction entails possible, or even probable differences among the perspectives of actors.

15   The several or many participants in an interactional course necessitate what Blumer termed the "alignment" (or "articulation") of their respective actions.

16   A major set of conditions for actors' perspectives, and thus their interactions, is their memberships in social worlds and subworlds. In contemporary societies, these memberships are often complex, overlapping, contrasting, conflicting, and not always apparent to the interactants.

17   Other conditions bearing on interactions can be thought of in terms of a conditional matrix, ranging from broader, more indirect conditions to narrower and more directly impacting ones. The specific relevance of conditions can be analyzed by means of tracking conditional paths.

(Continued)

TABLE 4.1 (Continued)

18	A useful fundamental distinction between classes of interactions is between the routine and the problematic. Problematic interactions involve "thought", or when more than one interactant is involved, then "discussion" also. An important aspect of problematic action can also be "debate" – disagreement over issues or their resolution. That is, an arena has been formed that will affect the future course of action.
19	Also problematic interactions frequently bring about a process of identity change that entails some degree of suffering and strangeness toward the selves of individuals or collectivities.

Source: Strauss (1993, pp. 23–44).

published 2 years after Strauss's death. In the preface, Corbin wrote that the writing of this edition was truly a collaborative effort. She and Strauss clarified and extended explanation of the first edition. They stressed that this was "not a recipe book to be applied to research in a step-by-step fashion" (p. xi).

Strauss and Corbin (1998) used the term microscopic examination of the data in place of the term line-by-line coding because the same analytic process can be applied to a word, sentence, or paragraph. More details on microscopic examination at the start of a study were included to help generate categories by a combination of open and axial coding. Micro conditions are narrow in scope while macro conditions are broad. Some important functions of microanalysis include helping researchers listen closely to what the participants said and how they said it. It helps prevent researchers from jumping to their own theoretical conclusions by considering the participants' interpretations. "The data are not being forced; they are being allowed to speak" (p. 65). Microanalysis uses procedures of comparative analysis. As data are broken down, labeled, and conceptualized, they are then grouped together to form categories. The properties and dimensions of the categories are developed. Properties are the characteristics or attributes of a category while dimensions specify the location of a property along a continuum.

Strauss and Corbin (1998) now specified criteria for choosing a central category. Many of them were already addressed by Glaser (1978) and Strauss (1987). Examples of the criteria included it being related to all other major categories; it appears frequently in the data; and it could explain variation as well as the main point of the data.

In the first edition, the name of the matrix was conditional matrix. Strauss and Corbin (1998) renamed this term to be the conditional/consequential matrix. The matrix was a device to help researchers organize and link concepts. Strauss and Corbin listed the ideas contained in their matrix:

1 Conditions/consequences do not stand alone.
2 The distinction between micro conditions and macro conditions is an artificial one.

3 Often conditions and consequences exist in clusters. They can be associated in various ways. They can vary with each other and also with related actions and interactions.

4 In addition, action/interaction can be carried out not only by individuals, but also by organizations and nations. Action and interaction occur in the structural context represented by conditions and consequences.

For the third edition of the *Basic of Qualitative Research: Techniques and Procedures for Developing Grounded Theory*, Corbin became the first author followed by Strauss (Corbin & Strauss, 2008). In the preface, Corbin shared that after Strauss' death, she tried to keep his vision in mind as she wrote this new edition. She was not developing an entirely new method but modernizing. "My aim is not to recreate his approach to analysis, but to combine what was good about the old editions with some aspects of contemporary thinking" (p. ix). Corbin explained that since the second edition of *Basics of Qualitative Research: Techniques and Procedures for Developing Grounded Theory*, a decade ago, she had been influenced by publications of contemporary feminists, constructivists, and postmodernists like Clarke (2005) and Charmaz (2006). Her current thinking was reflected in the third edition while keeping most of Strauss' basic approach to analysis.

Corbin agreed with the constructivists who viewed theories as constructed by researchers and their participants. This was a departure from Glaser and Strauss' (1967) positivist view that findings emerge from the data. In this third edition influenced by her nursing background, Corbin emphasized she wanted to develop knowledge that helps guide practice and bring about social justice and change. Corbin also supported feminists' beliefs that "we don't separate who we are as persons from the research and analysis that we do. Therefore, we must be self-reflective about how we influence the research process, and in turn, how it influences us" (Corbin & Strauss, 2008, p. 11).

Corbin stressed that just like in the previous editions of *Basics of Qualitative Research: Techniques and Procedures for Developing Grounded Theory*, the techniques and procedures included in this third edition are tools and not directives. The analytic process is flexible and guided by the interaction with data. Corbin and Strauss (2008) called for the need to frame the research question in a way that allows a researcher with enough flexibility to explore a topic under study in depth. The research question first should identify the topic area being studied and alert the reader to what about the specific topic that the researcher is interested in. As the study progresses, the research question becomes more refined and specific.

KEY POINTS IN STRAUSSIAN GROUNDED THEORY

- Strauss did not view grounded theory as a specific method but instead as a style of doing qualitative analysis.
- The research question begins as an open and broad one to allow flexibility in investigating the phenomenon being studied.
- In axial coding, data are put back together and connections are made between categories.
- Axial coding is accomplished by using the coding paradigm of conditions, action/interaction, and consequences.
- The analytic process is flexible since the techniques and procedures are only tools and not directives.
- In the third and fourth editions, Corbin's aim was not to recreate Strauss' approach to analysis but to combine what was good about the first two editions with some aspects of contemporary thinking like feminism.

Corbin (2013) explained that readers had some confusion about the first three versions of *Basics of Qualitative Research: Techniques and Procedures for Developing Grounded Theory* and assumed they were different books. Corbin assured readers that the methods described in each edition were essentially the same. The presentation was just different with each edition as the authors tried to clarify some areas of the method where readers had questions about. She also stressed that "just because the third edition does not refer to open, axial, and selective coding does not mean that these forms of coding are not part of the method. What is important is not what one calls the different types of coding but a basic understanding of the logic that underlies coding, which is to identify different levels of concepts and achieve integration of all of these to form theory" (pp. 171–172).

Corbin and Strauss (2015) published the fourth edition of *Basics of Qualitative Research: Techniques and Procedures for Developing Grounded Theory*. Chapters in the first part of this edition focus on the methodology and are "purposely abstract. They are not meant to demonstrate the method but to set the tone and provide the background for doing analysis" (p. 1). Their paradigm is an analytic tool to help researchers perform axial coding or coding around a category and organize and link concepts. There are three main components of the paradigm: Conditions, actions-interactions, and consequences or outcomes. She went on to stress that qualitative research is meant to be free flowing without a rigid approach to analysis.

Corbin and Strauss (2015, p. 160) updated their diagram of the conditional/consequential matrix to help analysts bring complexity into their analysis

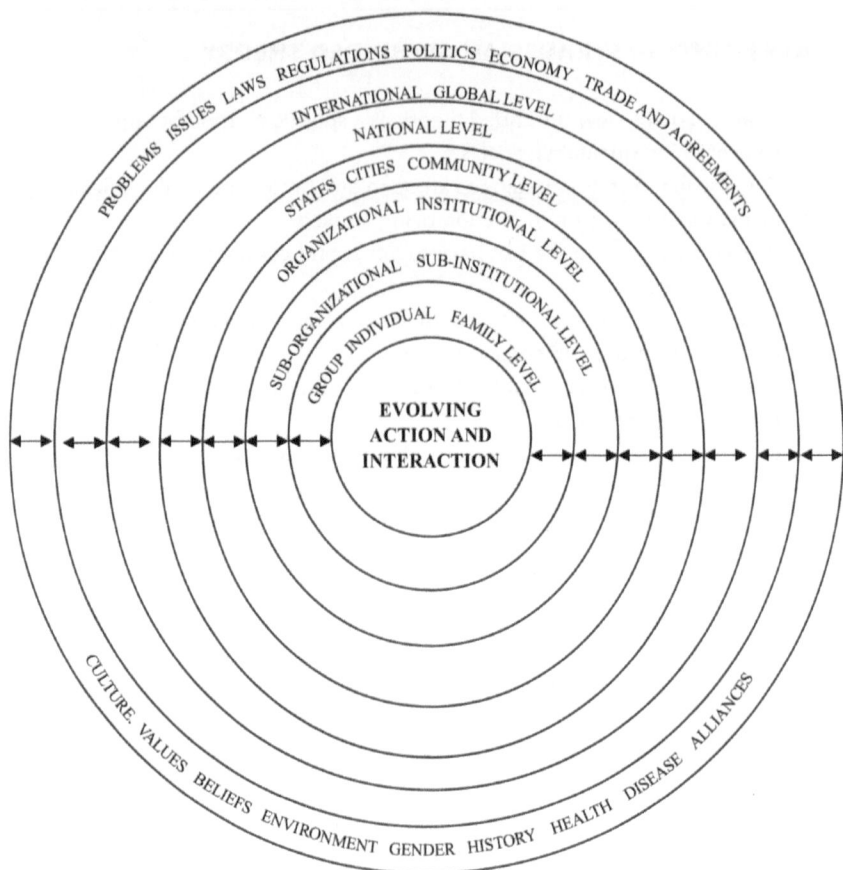

FIGURE 4.1 Corbin and Strauss Conditional/Consequential Matrix

Source: Reprinted with permission from Corbin and Strauss (2015, p. 163).

(Figure 4.1). It consists of a series of concentric and interconnected circles with arrows pointing both toward and away from the center. The arrows indicate where conditions and consequences intersect leading to a chain of events. The matrix directs researchers' attention to the following:

- Range of conditions and range of possible outcomes
- Complexity of the relationships between conditions, actions-interactions, and consequences
- Different actors, different perspectives
- Importance of micro and macro
- Putting it all together

Table 4.2 comprises the progression of Strauss and Corbin's publications.

TABLE 4.2 Progression of Strauss and Corbin's Publications

1973	**Schatzman and Strauss**
	Field Research: Strategies for a Natural Sociology
1987	**Strauss**
	Qualitative Analysis for Social Scientists
1990	**Strauss and Corbin**
	Basics of Qualitative Research: Techniques and Procedures for Developing Grounded Theory
1993	**Strauss**
	Continual Permutations of Action
1998	**Strauss and Corbin**
	Basics of Qualitative Research: Techniques and Procedures for Developing Grounded Theory (Second Edition)
2008	**Corbin and Strauss**
	Basics of Qualitative Research: Techniques and Procedures for Developing Grounded Theory (Third Edition)
2015	**Corbin and Strauss**
	Basics of Qualitative Research: Techniques and Procedures for Developing Grounded Theory (Fourth Edition)

Interdisciplinary Examples of Corbin and Strauss' Grounded Theory

From the discipline of Theology comes a grounded theory study using Corbin and Strauss' approach. Snow et al. (2023) investigated the experience of divine grace among 30 adult Protestant Christians. Open-ended questions in the interviews focused on the nature of the participants' relationship with God, what it means to be saved by grace, engagement with spiritual practice, and spiritual struggles. As the grounded theory developed, Snow et al. revised the interview questions based on emerging categories. Initial open coding, axial coding, and selective coding revealed that the participants often spoke of undeservedness of God's gift of grace. This notion of undeserved gifts included four dimensions of Protestant Christians' experience of grace: Salvific Grace, Ongoing Grace, Outcomes of Grace, and Obstacles to Grace. Salvific Grace included subthemes of focusing on the person and work of Jesus, God's character, and the significance of the afterlife. Ongoing Grace consisted of relationship with God and others, daily provisions, and use of metaphors. Outcomes of Grace involved being more caring for others and serving and obeying God. Obstacles to Grace focused on beliefs and attempts to earn or resist God's love.

From psychology, Kumar et al. (2023) conducted a grounded theory study of how university men envision themselves in the future. Using Corbin and Strauss' (2008) grounded theory approach, Kumar et al. developed the envisioning possible masculinities model (EPMM) using data from eight focus groups consisting of 49 university men in Canada. The researchers explained they chose Corbin and Strauss' method to grounded theory because of its emphasis on developing a theory for practical purposes. They used the Straussian analysis process of open, axial, and selective coding and the conditional/consequential matrix. The EPMM consisted of three major components: Current masculinity, systemic forces that contribute to how men envision their possible masculinities, and various components of possible masculinities. This data-driven theory indicated that the impact over time was subtle and gradual. There can be, however, critical incidents that can occur at different system levels of micro, meso, exo, and macrosystem levels.

Nurse researchers Michaels and Meeker (2024) undertook a grounded theory study using Corbin and Strauss's method to investigate family caregiving for older adults in rural areas. Fifteen family caregivers in two rural counties of New York state participated in the study. Two semi-structured interviews were conducted with each participant. Michaels and Meeker analyzed the data using open, axial, and selective coding. Results revealed that family care providers used a process of Orchestrating Care by three phases: Growing into Caregiving, Integrating Technology, and Using Networks. Growing into Caregiving involved acquiring caregiving skills and knowledge and developing coping strategies. Integrating Technology included gathering information, providing a safe and secure living situation, and promoting opportunities for socialization. Lastly, Utilizing Networks consisted of relying on relationships and confronting barriers.

In Sport and Exercise Sciences, Uzzell et al. (2024) utilized Corbin and Strauss' (2015) grounded theory approach to examine the process of high-performance swimmers in the United Kingdom to experience positive well-being while other swimmers struggled. Interviews were conducted via zoom with twenty-two current swimmers, five retired swimmers, eight coaches, and seven support staff. In addition to interviews, Uzzell attended numerous virtual meetings and social events with swimmers and coaches and observed training sessions and team meetings. Using open and axial coding, analysis revealed the core category of questioning or reaffirming swimmers' identity in response to performances during periods of change and uncertainty. The process started with being socialized at an early age into the sport. Next was the development of an exclusive swimmer identity as it became a central focus in their lives. The third phase included continually striving for performance improvements. Lastly, swimmers were able to effectively cope with change or uncertainty in their performance and identity.

In France Bertrand and Morvillers (2025) conducted a Straussian grounded theory study to explore psychiatric and mental health nurses' perceptions of patients with co-occurring psychiatric and substance use disorders in psychiatric settings. Participants were recruited at a public psychiatric hospital in Paris. Eleven psychiatric and mental health nurses participated in face-to-face interviews. Using Corbin and Strauss' (2015) data analysis method, open, axial, and selective coding were performed to identify the core category of waiting for a patient's will to change to emerge. This core category focused on the nurses' state of waiting for patients in psychiatric care while they concurrently asserted reluctance to change their substance use behavior. Bertrand and Morvillers' grounded theory adhered to Corbin and Strauss' paradigm model of conditions, action/interaction strategies, and consequences in their analysis and reporting of findings. Examples of conditions identified were nurses' confidence in their clinical abilities, and variations in the nurse-patient relationship. Nurses' action-interaction strategies focused on balancing the clinical and relational aspects of care. Nurses tried to preserve clinical stability and the quality of their relationship with patients while waiting for their patients to express their readiness for change. The consequence was collaboration through emergence of a patient's will to change.

End-of-Chapter Student Exercise

Conduct a cross-disciplinary search for the past 5 years using databases, such as PubMed, PsycINFO, ERIC, and Scopus, to locate studies using Corbin and Strauss' grounded theory approach. Select one study that interests you and use the following questions to guide your assessment of that study:

1 Did the researchers follow Corbin and Strauss' approach? If not, which aspects of their methodology were not followed?
2 What was the research question the researchers used to guide their study? Was it congruent with Corbin and Strauss' methodology?
3 Was the data analysis technique used appropriate for Corbin and Strauss' approach? Which types of coding did the researchers use in their analysis?
4 Did the researchers use the coding paradigm of conditions, context, action/interactional strategies, and consequences?
5 If you were to conduct this grounded theory study using Corbin and Strauss' approach, are there any aspects of it you would revise to strengthen its methodology?

References

Bertrand, E., & Morvillers, J. M. (2025). Nurses' perceptions of patients with co-occurring psychiatric and substance use disorders in psychiatric settings: A grounded theory study. *Journal of Advanced Nursing*. https://doi.org/10.1111/jan.16748

Charmaz, K. (2006). *Constructing grounded theory: A practical guide through qualitative analysis*. Sage.

Clarke, A. E. (2005). *Situational analysis: Grounded theory after the postmodern turn*. Sage.

Clarke, A. E., Friese, C., & Washburn, R. S. (2018). *Situational analysis: Grounded theory after the interpretive turn*. Sage.

Corbin, J. (2013). Strauss' grounded theory. In C. T. Beck (Ed.), *Routledge international handbook of qualitative nursing research* (pp. 169–182). Routledge.

Corbin, J., & Strauss, A. (2008). *Basics of qualitative research: Techniques and procedures for developing grounded theory* (3rd ed.). Sage.

Corbin, J., & Strauss, A. (2015). *Basics of qualitative research: Techniques and procedures for developing grounded theory* (4th ed.). Sage.

Glaser, B. G. (1978). *Theoretical sensitivity: Advances in the methodology of grounded theory*. Sociology Press.

Glaser, B. G., & Strauss, A. (1967). *The discovery of grounded theory: Strategies for qualitative research*. Aldine de Gruyter.

Kumar, R., Bedi, P., & Owin Lo, R. P. (2023). Possible masculinities: A grounded theory of how university men envision themselves in the future. *Qualitative Psychology, 10*(3), 435–451. https://doi.org/10.1037/qup0000261

Michaels, J. A., & Meeker, M. A. (2024). Orchestrating care: A grounded theory study of family caregiving for older adults in rural areas. *Qualitative Health Research, 34*(12), 1231–1242. https://doi.org/10.1177/10497323241236308

Schatzman, L., & Strauss, A. L. (1973). *Field research: Strategies for a natural sociology*. Prentice-Hall, Inc.

Snow, L. M., Hall, M. E. L., Hill, P. C., & Edwards, K. J. (2023). An undeserved gift from God: Conservative Christian experience of divine grace. *Journal of Psychology and Theology, 51*(4), 492–508. https://doi.org/10.1177/00916471231178875

Strauss, A., & Corbin, J. (1990). *Basics of qualitative research: Techniques and procedures for developing grounded theory*. Sage.

Strauss, A., & Corbin, J. (1998). *Basics of qualitative research: Techniques and procedures for developing grounded theory* (2nd ed.). Sage.

Strauss, A. L. (1987). *Qualitative analysis for social scientists*. Cambridge University Press.

Strauss, A. L. (1993). *Continual permutations of action*. Routledge.

Uzzell, K. S., Knight, C. J., Pankow, K., & Hill, D. M. (2024). Wellbeing in high-performance swimming: A grounded theory study. *Psychology of Sport and Exercise, 70*, 102557. https://doi.org/10.1016/j.psychsport.2023.102557

5

LEONARD SCHATZMAN AND BARBARA BOWERS' DIMENSIONAL ANALYSIS

Leonard Schatzman, a sociologist, was a student of Anselm Strauss at Indiana University and later became a colleague and published a book together, *Field Research: Strategies for a Natural Sociology* (Schatzman & Strauss, 1973). In that book Schatzman wrote a chapter on strategy for analyzing qualitative data. Schatzman (1991) firmed up his alternative approach to grounded theory which he named dimensional analysis. Schatzman learned about constant comparison from Strauss but in his approach, Schatzman wanted a broader way to analyze qualitative data to generate a theory. Instead of concentrating on a basic social psychological process, Schatzman wanted an approach to answer the question, "What all is going on?" Schatzman felt that Strauss' grounded theory did not address the complexity in analyzing qualitative data. He stressed that dimensionalizing permits a person to view things in their complexity and helps to compare one thing with another.

Schatzman (1991) did state that dimensional analysis "is generally informed by the core ideas and practices of grounded theory" (p. 303). He felt that additional analytical processes were needed besides comparative analysis. Schatzman's dimensional analysis is also based on pragmatism and symbolic interaction as Strauss' grounded theory is. Important aspects of natural analysis are considerations. Considerations or conjuring about a phenomenon focus on dimensions of an experience. Schatzman (1991, p. 309) explained that "the conjuring (calling out in oneself), assembly and configuration or patterning of situational components, conceived dimensionally, is analysis". Schatzman went on to state that the definition of a constructed situation is a theory of it. He considered Strauss' matrix of context, conditions, actions, and consequences in a wider view of providing a

DOI: 10.4324/9781032695563-5

structure that could totally frame or direct the perspective of analysis. The matrix was not just for coding. It was the cornerstone of analysis. Perspective was essential. "From perspective, in context, under conditions, specified actions, with consequences frame the story in terms of an explanatory logic" (Schatzman, 1991, p. 308). In analysis an understanding of all considerations involved in a phenomenon constitutes the whole of it. For each new aspect that is conjured, it, the whole, and the cognitive problem itself change in a continual process of analysis and definition. In dimensional analysis the methodological question is "What all is involved here?" (Schatzman, 1991, p. 310).

Schatzman called for accumulating a "critical mass of dimensions" before they are assigned to positions in the matrix. Dimensions can be converted to a perspective which helps control dimensional assignment to positions in the matrix such as, condition, process, and consequences. For Schatzman the most fundamental operation in qualitative data analysis was discovering significant "classes of things, persons, and events and the properties which characterize them" (Schatzman & Strauss, 1973, p. 110). He described three types of classes: Common, special, and theoretical. Next these classes are named and linked to one another with propositional statements. After researchers identify a key linkage or overriding pattern or story line, they can be selective in which classes they need to focus on. Researchers move back and forth between collecting data and analyzing data.

The other analytic processes required to conduct dimensional analysis included (1) conjuring, calling up dimensions and characteristics, (2) assigning relative value to each dimension to help decide which dimensions to include or not in generating a theory, and (3) making inferences about the conjured dimensions (Bowers & Schatzman, 2009; 2021). In Schatzman's approach to grounded theory, he suggested that comparative analysis be delayed until a researcher had a large number of dimensions generated from the data.

When designating dimensions in data, prior assumptions of the researcher lead to recognizing which dimensions are relevant. Schatzman believed that research analysis is fundamentally the same as natural analysis; what we all do every day. Dimensional analysis focuses on how situations are defined. In dimensional analysis Schatzman (1991) called for selecting the dimensions that are relevant to the situation and organizing them. Their analytic attributes relevant or irrelevant to implicit or explicit dimensions are focused on. Which dimensions are central to the situation and which are less important are considered. It is both context and perspective that impact which dimensions are most salient in defining the situation. Schatzman used Strauss' matrix not for coding but in terms of providing a total framework or methodological perspective for analysis. His explanatory matrix is the overarching framework of Schatzman's analytic process.

After 1991, Schatzman did not publish further on his own about dimensional analysis. His graduate students continued publications using his method that he guided them on. Barbara Bowers, a nursing PhD, published with Schatzman (Bowers & Schatzman, 2009; 2021) and provided more specifics of his dimensional analysis method. Kools et al. (1996) studied with Schatzman for more than 3 years and provided a research exemplar to illustrate dimensional analysis.

The perspectives of a researcher and participants and context are integrated into defining a situation. The meaning of a situation is constructed by the process of dimensionalizing (Caron & Bowers, 2000). Researcher and informants' perspectives direct the analysis and determine which dimensions are important. Researchers' past experiences and knowledge (recognition/recall) are an integral part of dimensional analysis. They help recognize relevant dimensions. When researchers do not take their perspectives into account when they analyze data, they can misinterpret the data (Bowers & Schatzman, 2021). "Recognition/recall involves the use of prior/received theory, often unwittingly to conceptualize data while mistakenly attributing that conceptualization to analysis of the object of interest" (p. 122). Schatzman warned that recognition/recall can deter analysis preventing the researcher from conjuring new dimensions and their properties. Findings emerge from the interaction between the researcher's perspective and the data to be analyzed.

KEY POINTS IN SCHATZMAN & BOWERS' DIMENSIONAL ANALYSIS

- Strauss' matrix of context, conditions, action, and consequences was not just for coding in dimensional analysis but was the cornerstone of analysis of the complexity of a situation.
- Perspective is essential.
- Researcher and participants' perspectives direct the analysis and determine which dimensions are important.
- Schatzman wanted a broader way to analyze qualitative data to generate a theory.
- Schatzman's approach answers the question, "What all is going on?"

Bowers' (1987) study on intergenerational caregiving provided specific examples of her and Schatzman's dimensional analysis method. Thirty-three adult caregivers of their aging parents comprised the sample. Theoretical sampling was based on comparisons between cognitive and physical impairments and various living arrangements. The main source of data was by means of interviews. An example of an early interview question was "What is it like to be a caregiver of one's parent?" (p. 24). Later interview questions became more focused on consequences of failed caregiving and strategies for invisible caregiving. These interview questions were:

- How does one care for an aging parent while preventing the parent from discovering that he or she is being cared for?
- How does this goal influence interactions with other offspring, other relatives, or health care providers?
- What strategies are used to respond to the parent who perceives that he or she is being cared for?
- Under what conditions are parents not upset about being cared for by offspring? How would this affect strategies for caregiving?

(Bowers, 1987, p. 24)

By means of dimensional analysis, Bowers learned that the work of caring for an aging parent was mainly invisible. Five conceptually distinct but empirically overlapping categories of the process of caregiving were revealed: Anticipatory, preventive, supervisory, instrumental, and protective caregiving. Bowers identified three strategies for protective caregiving: (1) To protect the parent from awareness of an event, (2) to protect the parent from awareness of the meaning of a situation, and (3) to continually reconstruct the meaning of an event. In Bowers' (1987) grounded theory, she discovered that only one of the categories of caregiving involved hands-on caregiving behaviors or tasks. The other four categories involved invisible behaviors that were not observable behaviors.

Table 5.1 consists of the progression of Schatzman and Bowers' publications.

TABLE 5.1 Progression of Schatzman and Bowers' Publications of Dimensional Analysis

Year	Author/Title
1973	**Schatzman and Strauss**
	Field Research: Strategies for a Natural Sociology
1991	**Schatzman**
	Dimensional Analysis: Notes on an Alternative Approach to Grounding of Theory in Qualitative Research
2009	**Bowers and Schatzman**
	Dimensional Analysis in Morse et al.
	Developing Grounded Theory: The Second Generation
2021	**Bowers and Schatzman**
	Dimensional Analysis in Morse et al.
	Developing Grounded Theory: The Second Generation Revisited

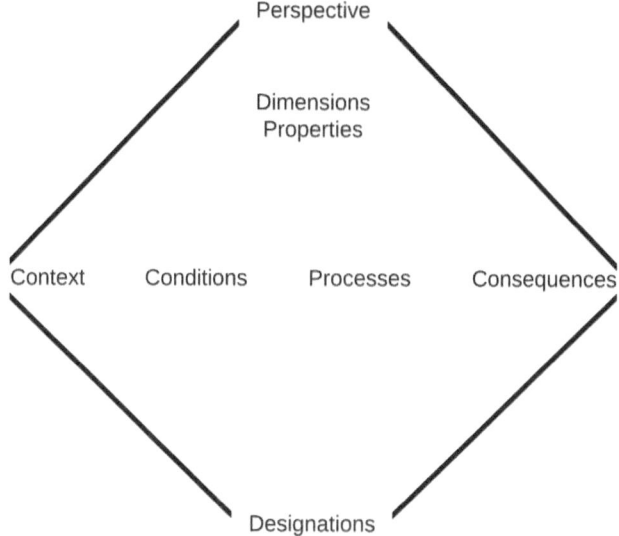

FIGURE 5.1   Schatzman's Explanatory Matrix

Source: Reprinted with permission from Kools et al. (1996, p. 318).

From the discipline of nursing, Kools et al. (1996) closely studied dimensional analysis under Schatzman and provided a figure to illustrate his explanatory matrix (Figure 5.1). Context refers to the environment or setting where dimensions occur. Conditions are the most relevant dimensions. Processes are the actions or interactions that are driven by specific conditions. Lastly consequences are the outcomes of specific interactions. As analysis continues, the researcher selects the central dimension which provides the greatest explanation of the relationship among dimensions. The chosen central dimension is now referred to as the perspective and is used to organize the other relevant dimensions for the developing theory. Dimensions that are more peripheral to the perspective are identified as context.

Kools et al. (1996) stated that once the organizing perspective is chosen, theoretical sampling continues to aid the researcher in solidifying the relationships among dimensions and stimulates integration. Kools et al. (1996, p. 320) provided another figure that helps illustrate Schatzman's dimensional analysis. Figure 5.2 shows the steps a researcher takes to select the perspective.

Interdisciplinary Examples of Dimensional Analysis

Altman et al. (2019) from the discipline of nursing conducted a dimensional analysis of experiences of women of color interacting with health care providers in pregnancy and birth in the United States. The researchers interviewed

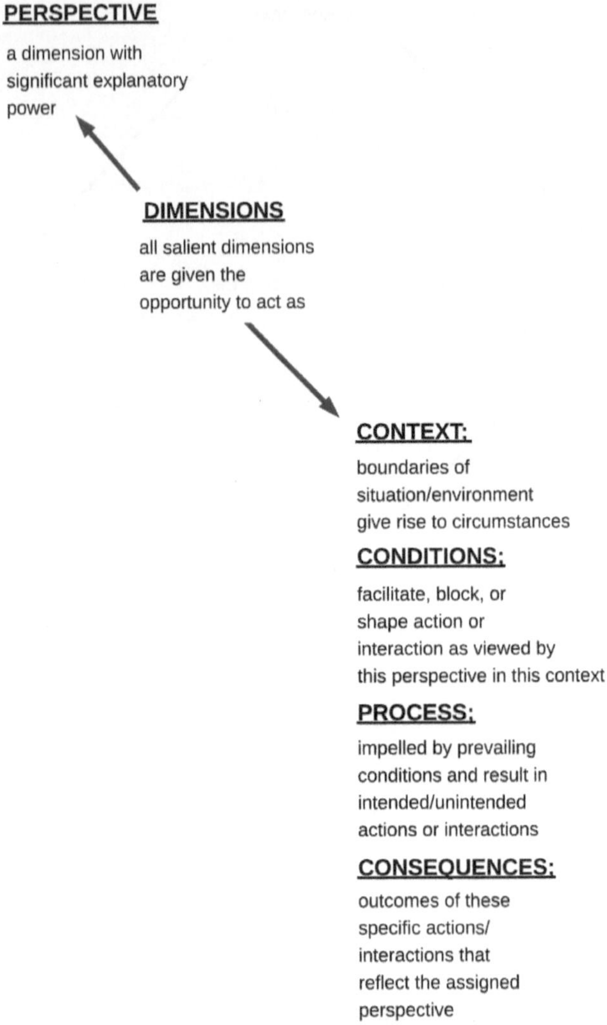

PERSPECTIVE

a dimension with
significant explanatory
power

DIMENSIONS

all salient dimensions
are given the
opportunity to act as

CONTEXT:

boundaries of
situation/environment
give rise to circumstances

CONDITIONS:

facilitate, block, or
shape action or
interaction as viewed by
this perspective in this context

PROCESS:

impelled by prevailing
conditions and result in
intended/unintended
actions or interactions

CONSEQUENCES:

outcomes of these
specific actions/
interactions that
reflect the assigned
perspective

FIGURE 5.2   Steps a Researcher Takes to Select a Perspective in Dimensional Analysis

Source: Reprinted with permission from Kools et al. (1996, p. 320).

22 women of color who were between 6 weeks and 1 year postpartum. Transcripts were analyzed using dimensional analysis. Altman et al. organized
codes within Schatzman's (1991) matrix that included a dominant perspective and related context, conditions, processes, and consequences. Multiple
dimensions or perspectives were identified to determine the dominant perspective with the most explanatory power of interactions of women of color
with clinicians while seeking care for pregnancy and birth. The dominant
perspective chosen was power and privilege in patient-provider information

exchange. Obstetrical clinicians had control over the information they shared and "packaged" information to exert power over women of color's capacity to participate in decision-making about their own care in pregnancy and birth. The manner in which information was shared could either empower or disempower women of color. Two conditions influenced the information exchange. The first condition was establishing relationships with providers that can lead to improved information exchange. The second condition focused on the visible or acknowledged sources of privilege and marginalization that women of color brought with them into their interactions with obstetrical clinicians. Contextual factors that influenced patient-clinician interactions included bias and judgment, health care system barriers, and power in context. Consequences of clinicians' control over information resulted in a power dynamic that decreased women of color's ability to maintain autonomy and make health care decisions for themselves regarding their childbearing care.

In her dissertation from the discipline of nursing, Whitney (2020) utilized dimensional analysis to uncover the experience and circumstances under which clinicians moralize substance use in maternal-child symbiosis. She wanted to investigate "What all is involved" with moralizing substance use during maternal-child symbiosis. Whitney used theoretical sampling with snowball sampling to recruit 15 participants in her study. Primary data sources were interviews and investigator's research memos. Whitney also created graphic memos to help her visualize the dimensions of data analysis. Using constant comparative techniques, she developed an explanatory matrix where she organized theoretical codes by conceptual categories of perspective, context, conditions, processes, and consequences. Dimensional analysis revealed one main contextual dimension of unacceptability uncertainty. The perspective involved was "Am I a good enough clinician?" In unacceptable uncertainty the clinicians needed to plan a patient's care based on information they perceive to be uncertain. The sole conditional dimension that influenced the process involved in moralizing substance use during maternal-child symbiosis was the truthfulness factor. The condition of the truthfulness factor involved clinicians feeling that parents do not trust them to be "good enough" at providing care. Moral energy reflex was the process involved, and it encompassed the actions and interactions of moralizing substance use during maternal-child symbiosis. It consisted of the primary steps of internalizing moral energy and redirecting moral energy. The secondary steps involved sympathization and moralization. The consequence identified by Whitney was reflection on redirection.

The purpose of Yu and Bowers' (2020) study was to develop a conceptual model that described the experience of immigrant women's postpartum distress, and the dimensions involved in their response to this distress. Their sample consisted of 22 Chinese immigrant women who had given birth within the last 3 years. Using constant comparison, Yu and Bowers immediately began dimensionalizing their data from face to face interviews with the participants using Schatzman's grounded theory approach. Based on the dimensions of self and loss, they developed a conceptual model of grayscaling and reviving the psychological self. Grayscaling the psychological self described the process of experiencing distress in response to the dimensions of loss. Reviving the psychological self entailed the process of resolving distress and regaining or transforming their psychological self. The following dimensions of self evolved across time from the old self to current self to potential self: Psychological, physical, social, and spiritual. While simultaneously transitioning from woman to mother and also from native to foreign Chinese immigrants, women faced many significant losses to their psychological self. This grounded theory model provides pathways the participants used to respond to these loses and resolve distress.

End-of-Chapter Student Exercise

Using various databases, conduct a cross-disciplinary search for any Schatzman and Bowers' dimensional analysis studies published in the past 5 years. Choose one study that interests you and comment on its methodology using the following questions as a guide:

- Did the study follow Schatzman and Bowers' dimensional analysis methodology? If not, what aspects of their approach were not followed?
- Did the researchers use Schatzman's explanatory matrix of content, conditions, actions/process, and consequences to direct their analysis?
- What dimensions and their characteristics were identified in the situation under study?
- Did the researchers assign relative values to the identified dimensions to decide which ones to include in their grounded theory study?
- Did the researchers explain how they took their perspectives of past experiences and knowledge into account during analysis and interpretation of data?
- If you were to conduct this dimensional analysis using Schatzman and Bowers' approach, are there any aspects of it you would change to strengthen its methodology?

References

Altman, M. R., Oseguera, T., McLemore, M. R., Kantrowitz-Gordon, I., Franck, L. S., & Lyndon, A. (2019). Information and power: Women of color's experiences interacting with health care providers in pregnancy and birth. *Social Science and Medicine*, *238*, 112491. https://doi.org/10.1016/j.socscimed.2019.112491

Bowers, B. J. (1987). Intergenerational caregiving: Adult caregivers and their aging parents. *Advances in Nursing Science*, *9*(2), 20–31.

Bowers, B. J., & Schatzman, L. (2009). Dimensional analysis. In J. M. Morse, P. N. Stern, J. Corbin, B. Bowers, K. Charmaz, & A. E. Clarke (Eds.), *Developing grounded theory: The second generation* (pp. 86–106). Left Coast Press.

Bowers, B. J., & Schatzman, L. (2021). Dimensional analysis. In J. M. Morse, B. J. Bowers, K. Charmaz, A. E. Clarke, J. Corbin, C. J. Porr, & P. N. Stern (Eds.), *Developing grounded theory: The second generation revisited* (pp. 111–129). Routledge.

Caron, C. D., & Bowers, B. J. (2000). Methods and application of dimensional analysis: A contribution to concept and knowledge development in nursing. In B. L. Rogers & K. A. Knafl (Eds.), (pp. 285–319). *Concept development in nursing.* W.B. Saunders Company.

Kools, S., McCarthy, M., Durham, R., & Robrecht, L. (1996). Dimensional analysis: Broadening the conception of grounded theory. *Qualitative Health Research, 6*(3), 312–330.

Schatzman, L. (1991). Dimensional analysis: Notes on an alternative approach to the grounding of theory in qualitative research. In D. Maines (Ed.), *Social organization and social process: Essays in honor of Anslem Strauss* (pp. 303–314). Aldine de Gruyter.

Schatzman, L., & Strauss, A. L. (1973). *Field research: Strategies for a natural sociology.* Prentice-Hall, Inc.

Whitney, C. E. (2020). *Moralizing substance use in maternal-child symbiosis: An emergent fit dimensional analysis.* Dissertation. University of Pennsylvania.

Yu, Z., & Bowers, B. (2020). "Everything is grayscaled": Immigrant women's experiences of postpartum distress. *Qualitative Health Research, 30*(9), 1445–1461. https://doi.org/10.1177/1049732320914868

6

ADELE CLARKE'S SITUATIONAL ANALYSIS

As a second-generation grounded theorist, Adele Clarke, a sociologist, (2005) modified her grounded theory approach after the interpretive turn. This turn happened in the late 20th century where shifts occurred in social sciences, humanities, and professional schools toward more postmodern, poststructural and interpretive approaches to qualitative research. The interpretive turn is based on the premise that human inquiry is understanding the human experience from within a specific situation. Clarke et al.'s (2018) situational analysis is based on both Straussian grounded theory (Strauss, 1987; Strauss & Corbin, 1990; 1998) and Charmaz's (2014) constructivist grounded theory. It shares their roots of pragmatism and social interaction. In her grounded theory approach, Clarke included nonhuman entities in the situation. Nonhuman entities/things are components of social interaction theory (Blumer, 1969). Glaser and Strauss' (1967) and Glaser's (1978) grounded theory focused on discovering one basic social process but in situational analysis Clarke replaced this by focusing on the situation under study as the key unit of analysis. Clarke et al. (2018) designed their grounded theory approach to remove some of what they termed positivist recalcitrances in grounded theory. One of these was a lack of reflexivity. They pointed out that the addition of intentional reflexivity to the research process is an epistemological break from Glaserian grounded theory. Clarke et al. urged reflexivity as a part of the research process and a requisite for good data analysis.

In situational analysis the researchers making several kinds of analytic maps help the analyst understand the dense complexities of a particular situation (Clarke, 2021). The four kinds of maps needed to analyze the situation under study are:

- Situational maps which include all the elements in the situation, both human and nonhuman.

DOI: 10.4324/9781032695563-6

- Relational maps which focus on the relations among all the elements identified in the situational map.
- Social worlds/arenas maps detail all the collective actors such as organizations, institutions, and their areas of action in the situation. Arenas are the sites where social worlds meet. Clarke elaborated on Strauss' social worlds/arenas theory.
- Positional maps address positions taken and not taken in discourses included in the situation under study. These maps help portray the various positions held on key issues in the situation.

Situational analysis extended Straussian grounded theory. Strauss and Corbin in their grounded theory included a conditional matrix to help frame grounded theory to include structural conditions. Strauss and Corbin's matrix helped researchers to envision the conditions and contexts under which an action occurred. Structural conditions were viewed as context around the central action. Clarke developed new approaches to focus on the broader situation as the phenomenon in her situational matrix. Now the conditions of the situation are in the situation. There is no longer context. The conditional elements of the situation are no longer viewed as surrounding it. "They are in it" (Clarke, 2021, p. 231). Clarke's fundamental assumption of structural analysis is that "everything in the situation both co-constitutes and affects most everything else in the situation in some way" (p. 232).

Situational analysis is an extension of grounded theory method and shares common roots and assumptions with classic grounded theory. There is, however, a totally different form of analysis from Glaser and Strauss' (1967) grounded theory where action and interaction and processes take center stage. Clarke et al.'s (2018) situational analysis focuses on relationality where mapping and memoing the ecologies of relations occur among the various elements in a situation (situational maps), the different social groups and sites (social worlds/arenas maps), and discourses in the situation (positional maps). In Clarke's extension of grounded theory method, she integrated discourse analysis (Foucault, 1973) of extant materials like visual, historical, and narrative, which are present in the situation being studied.

KEY POINTS IN CLARKE'S SITUATIONAL ANALYSIS

- Instead of focusing on discovery of a basic social process, the situation under study is the key unit of analysis.
- Data analysis involves making four maps: Situational, relational, social worlds/arenas, and positional.

- Clark includes nonhuman entities in the situation under study.
- An "ambitious literature review" provides an invaluable help to researchers defining their research question.
- Social worlds are collective groupings of different sizes which have shared commitment and resources toward reaching their goals.
- Positional maps are used to analyze discursive materials in the situation under study.

To start, Clarke et al.'s (2018) approach includes the researchers' own experiences of the phenomenon being studied. Also, what she called "ambitious literature review" (p. 112) will be an invaluable help as researchers refine their research questions and identify the gap in the knowledge base that the situational analysis will fill. Memoing from the very beginning is essential.

Analysis begins with researchers creating a messy situational map. Included here are all possible analytically important human and nonhuman, material, discursive elements that occur in a situation. Figure 6.1 is an abstract situational messy map. Some examples of key questions a researcher should ask at this stage of analysis are "What nonhuman things really matter

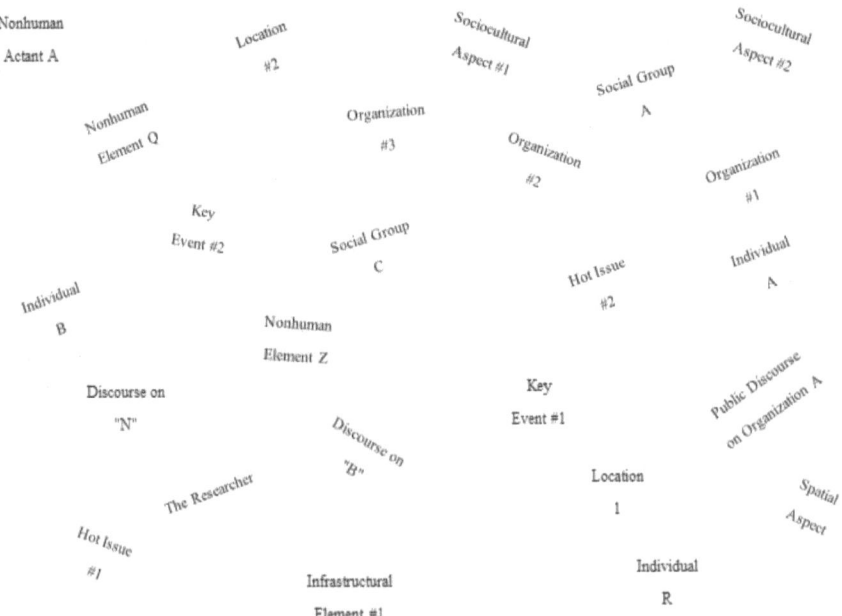

FIGURE 6.1   Abstract Situational Map: Messy Version

Source: Reprinted with permission from Clarke et al. (2018, p. 128).

Individual Human Elements/Actors	Nonhuman Elements/ Actants
e.g., key individuals and significant (unorganized) people in the situation, including the researcher (s)	e.g., technologies; material infrastructures; specialized information and/or knowledges; material "things"
Collective Human Elements/Actors	Implicated/Silent Actors/Actants
e.g., particular groups; specific organizations	As found in the situation
Discursive Constructions of Individual and/or Collective Human Actors	Discursive Constructions of Nonhuman Actants
As found in the situation	As found in the situation
Political/Economic Elements	Sociocultural/Symbolic Elements
e.g., the state; particular industry/ies; local/regional/global orders; political parties; NGOs; politicized issues	e.g., religion; race; sexuality; gender; ethnicity; nationality; logos; icons; other visual and/or aural symbols
Temporal Elements	Spatial Elements
e.g., historical, seasonal, crises, and/or trajectory aspects	e.g., spaces in the situation, geographical aspects, local, regional, national, global, spatial issues
Major Issues/Debates (Usually Contested)	Related Discourses (Historical, Narrative, and/or Visual)
as found in the situation; and see positional map	e.g., normative expectations of actors, actants, and/or other specified elements; moral/ethical elements; mass media and other
Other Kinds of Elements	

FIGURE 6.2   Abstract Situational Map: Ordered Version

Source: Reprinted with permission from Clarke et al. (2018, p. 131).

in this situation of inquiry? To whom or what do they matter?" (Clarke et al., 2018, p. 129). Situational maps can help identify what is taken for granted in the situation under study. Clarke et al. (2018) stressed that researchers need to include themselves in a situational map by engaging in reflexivity.

Messy situational maps are revised across the research project. Using a messy map as data, another situational map can be created, this time, an ordered version. Figure 6.2 is an example of an abstract situational map: Ordered version. Clarke et al. (2018) made clear that situational maps are not conceptual or analytic diagrams based on grounded theory codes. They involve a very different type of analysis to help lay out the main elements of the situation being studied.

Relational analyses are done within situational maps. Here questions are focused on the relations among the various elements in the messy situational map. Researchers can take each element in turn and create a relational map where the lines are drawn between that element and the relations between other elements (Figure 6.3). What is the nature of the relationship the lines indicate? Researchers can create as many relational maps as necessary to focus on one element at a time.

Next social worlds/arenas maps are created. Social worlds are collective groupings of different sizes which have shared commitment and resources toward reaching their goals. Arenas are concerns around particular issues in the multiple social worlds. Key questions at this stage of analysis focus on "Who cares about which issues and what do they want to do about them?" (Clarke et al., 2018, p. 148). Clarke et al. provided a social worlds/arenas toolbox

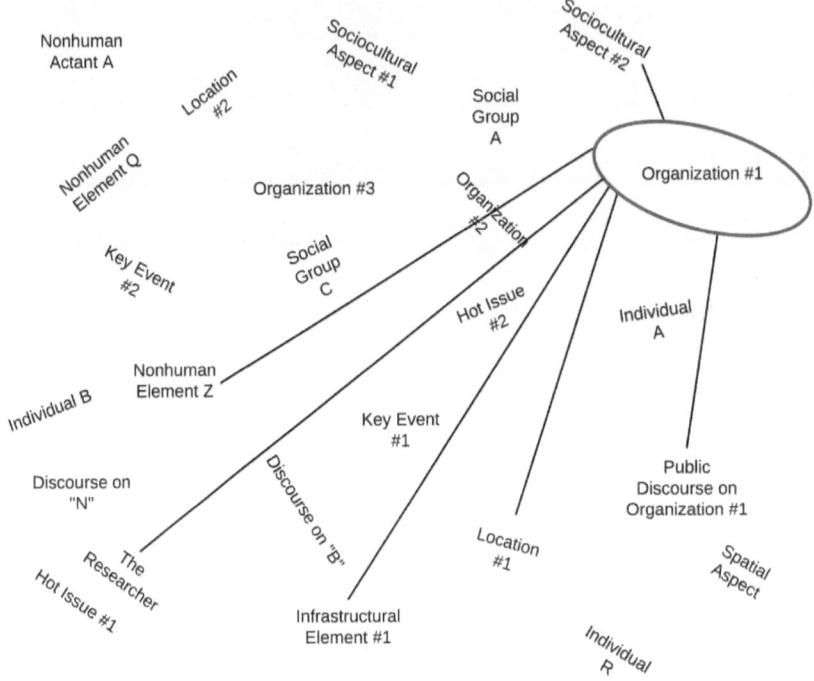

FIGURE 6.3 Abstract Relational Map: Focus on Organization # 1

Source: Reprinted with permission from Clarke et al. (2018, p. 139).

researchers can use to help create and analyze social worlds/arenas maps. Examples of this toolbox include share ideologies, particular sites, more formal organizations, work objects, and discourses. In these maps the focus is on social action by committed collectivities. Social worlds/arenas maps can be developed once a researcher has gathered some data and is starting to get a handle on the situation being studied. Figure 6.4 is an abstract map of social worlds in arenas. Clarke et al. (2018) emphasized that in this map the dotted lines represent the porous nature of the social worlds' boundaries and those of the arenas. When creating social worlds/arenas maps, researchers need to ask these research questions: "What are the patterns of collective commitment creating the social worlds operating here? Are there groups with shared interests and stakes?" (Clarke et al., 2018, p. 155).

In situational analysis, positional maps are used to analyze discursive materials in the situation. Data from fieldwork, interviews, participant observation, and documents are used to set out the main positions taken on issues in the situation under study. Positional maps focus on discourse analysis. Positions are not analyzed to how they are associated with groups or institutions. Positions taken or not taken are instead viewed in discourse. Figure 6.5 presents an abstract positional map. A question for researchers to include is:

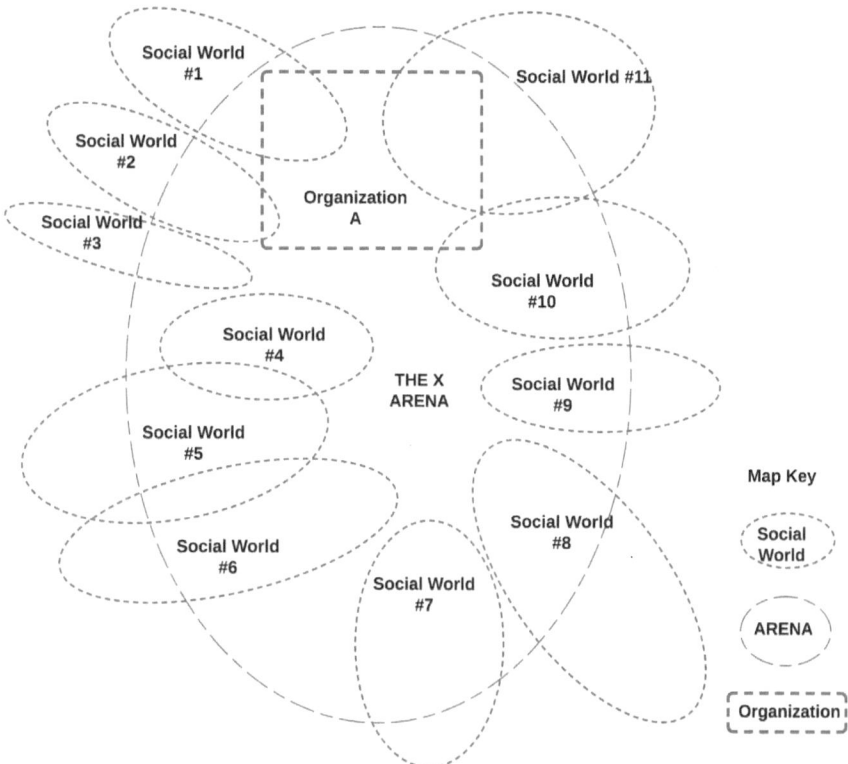

FIGURE 6.4   Abstract Map of Social Worlds in Arenas

Source: Reprinted with permission from Clarke et al. (2018, p. 152).

What are the issues debated here? Multiple positional maps may be needed. The researcher selects two related axes at a time which can portray the debated issues on a specific issue within the situation. Creating positional maps can help researchers see positions that are not taken in the data. As Clarke et al. (2018) suggested, "positional maps allow silences to be made to speak" (p. 172).

In addition to reflexivity, Clarke et al. (2018) in their situational analysis tried to revise some other positivist holdovers from Glaser and Strauss' (1967) and Glaser's (1978) grounded theory. Some of these positivist recalcitrances included a researcher should be "invisible", meaning a researcher should not co-construct the findings with the participants nor incorporate their positionality in their research. In the epilogue of their book, Clarke et al. (2018) stressed that "Situational analysis is deeply reflexive. It acknowledges the embodiment and situatedness of researchers and their positionality grounded in the research" (p. 358).

Table 6.1 consists of the progression of Clarke et al.'s situational analysis publications.

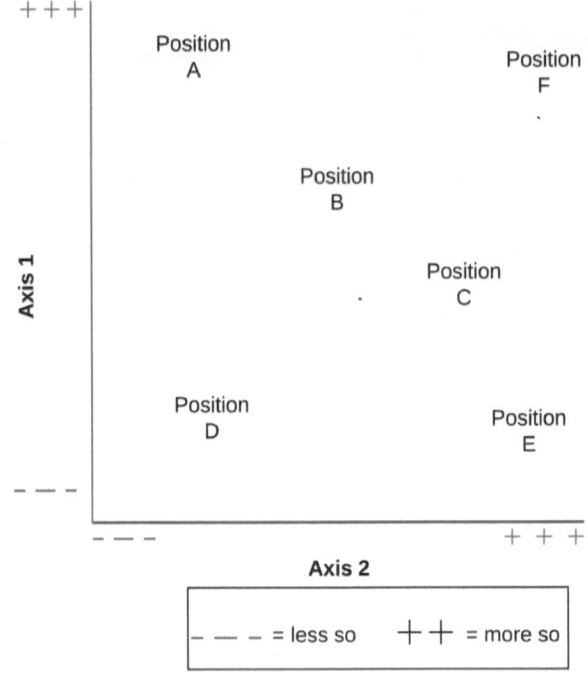

FIGURE 6.5 Abstract Positional Map

Source: Reprinted with permission from Clarke et al. (2018, p. 167).

TABLE 6.1 Progression of Clarke's Situational Analysis Publications

Year	Author/Title
2005	**Clarke** Situational Analysis: Grounded Theory after the Postmodern Turn
2009	**Clarke** From Grounded Theory to Situational Analysis: What's New? Why? How? in Morse et al. Developing Grounded Theory: The Second Generation
2015	**Clarke, Friese, and Washburn** Situational Analysis in Practice: Mapping Research with Grounded Theory
2018	**Clarke, Friese, and Washburn** Situational Analysis: Grounded Theory after Interpretative Turn (2nd Edition)
2021	**Clarke** From Grounded Theory to Situational Analysis: What's New? Why? How? in Morse et al. Developing Grounded Theory: The Second Generation Revisited
2022	**Clarke, Friese, Washburn** Situational Analysis in Practice: Mapping Relationalities across Disciplines (2nd Edition)

Interdisciplinary Examples of Situational Analysis

Beard and Johnson (2024) conducted a situational analysis of how nursing educators create psychological safety in the classroom. The aim of their study was to uncover the elements in the situation of a nursing classroom and institutional practices that connect to create psychological safety. Situational analysis facilitated constructing maps to help analysis by visualizing connections among both animate and inanimate factors in the situation under study (Clarke, 2005). The sample consisted of 16 nursing faculty with 5 or more years teaching experience and faculty with classroom teaching responsibilities. Semi-structured interviews yielded data that Beard and Johnson used to make their situational maps. A messy map displayed initial prominent elements and a relational map depicted the connections among the elements (Figure 6.6). An ordered map displayed initial categories which included protecting feelings, setting the stage, inviting students in, being a nurse/teacher, classroom/technology, documents, and objects. The grounded theory of psychological safety in the nursing classroom included the following various elements that shaped the situation of classroom learning environment: Allowing wrongness, reading the room, and leveling the balance. Analysis revealed the animate and inanimate objects in the nursing classroom were the faculty behaviors, the classroom space, and objects. The relationship between faculty behavior and how they used themselves to create a safe space revealed the situation where students' thinking and learning were prioritized over the

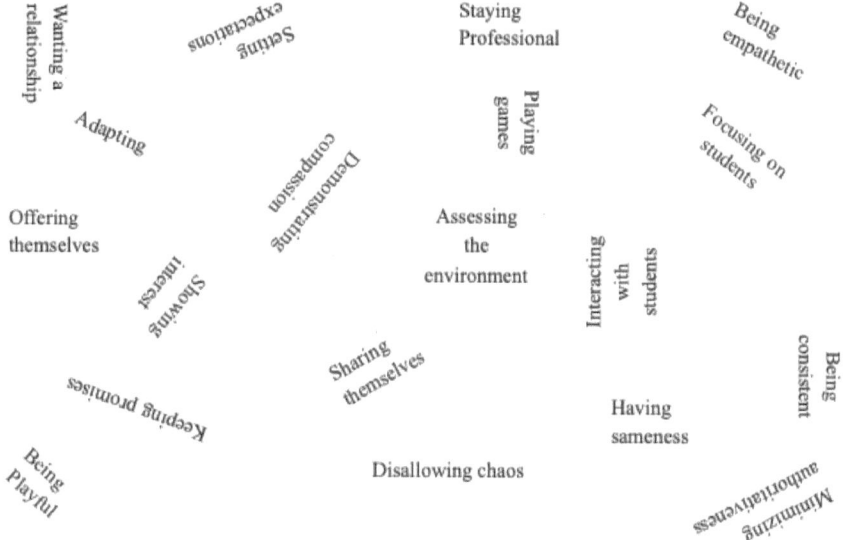

FIGURE 6.6   Initial Messy Map Displaying Preeminent Patterns

Source: Reprinted with permission from Beard & Johnson (2024, pp. 157–163).

correctness of their answers. The classroom space was also important that permitted faculty to roam among students giving faculty cues to read the room. Objects included documents and games that helped create psychological safety in the learning environment.

From the disciplines of gender studies, sociology, and physiotherapy, Öhman et al. (2023) conducted a situational analysis of Swedish elderly care. Their aim was to examine the perspectives of healthcare providers on professional knowledge development and evidence-based practice in their organizations. The sample consisted of 17 healthcare professionals: Five registered nurses, six physical therapists, and six occupational therapists. Fourteen participants were women and three were men. All were interviewed on site. Based on Clarke et al.'s (2018) situational analysis approach, Öhman et al. purposely selected a variety of healthcare organizations including public and private institutions, nursing homes, rehabilitation centers for the elderly, and geriatric hospitals. Swedish elderly care was considered the social world and the social arena, the situation being studied. Öhman et al. (2023) focused on positional maps illustrating various professional positions in relation to knowledge development in elderly care organizations. Situational analysis revealed three different professional discursive positions which are portrayed in the positional map along a continuum of approaches to knowledge development on one axis and a continuum of organizational factors on another axis (Figure 6.7). Position 1 represents

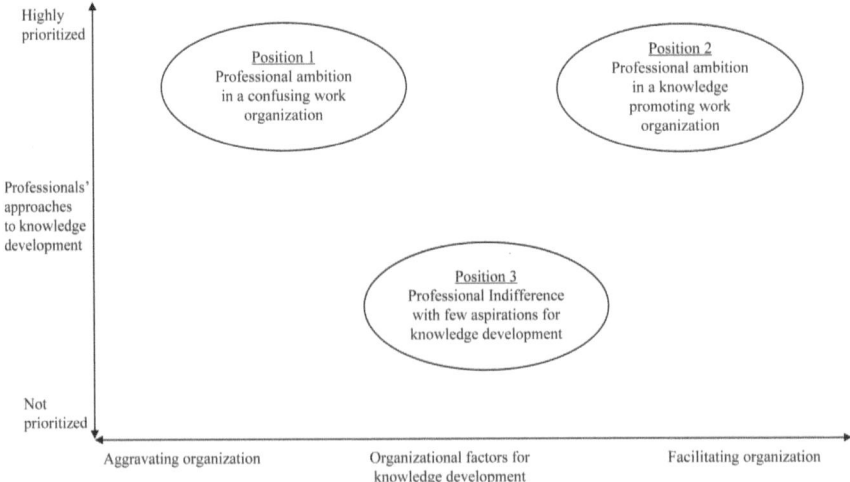

FIGURE 6.7 Positional Map of Professionals' Approaches to, and Organizational factor for, Knowledge Development and Evidence Based Practice in Elderly Care

Source: Reprinted with permission from Öhman et al. (2023, p. 999).

professional ambition toward evidence-based practice in a confusing work organization. Position 2 includes professional ambition in a knowledge-promoting work organization. Position 3 represents professional indifference with few aspirations for knowledge development. Situational analysis helped identify enabling and hindering factors in Swedish elderly care associated with professional knowledge development, continuing education, and evidence-based practice.

From palliative medicine, Wiesner et al. (2024) conducted a situational analysis of professionals' experiences and needs caring for parents who continued pregnancy after a life-limiting prenatal diagnosis in Germany. Semi-structured interviews were conducted online with 18 professionals from 12 different services. The sample included eight physicians, three midwives, two nurses, one pregnancy counselor, one grief counselor, one chaplain, one clinical psychologist, and one undertaker. Professionals experienced collateral beauty in providing perinatal palliative care despite all the suffering and grief. Collateral beauty referred to humble attitude, gratitude, and professional growth. Findings also revealed that professionals faced insufficient structures and inter-institutional collaboration. Wiesner et al. constructed a social arena map that included all the involved actors in a perinatal palliative care setting identified in their interviews.

End-of-Chapter Student Exercise

Conduct a cross-disciplinary search for grounded theory studies published in the past 5 years using situational analysis. Select one study that interests you and comment on its methodology using the following questions:

1 How well did the researchers describe Clarke et al.'s situational analysis research design? Were any essential elements of their methodology missing?
2 In their data analysis did the researchers make the four kinds of maps that are involved in situational analysis? Were figures of these maps included in the article to help visualize the findings? If not all four maps were included, which maps were? Situational, relational, social worlds/arenas, and/or positional?
3 Did the researchers identify any nonhuman entities in the situation under study?
4 What social worlds were involved in the situation being studied?
5 Were discursive materials analyzed in a positional map of the situation under study?
6 If you were to conduct this situational analysis study using Clarke et al.'s approach, are there any aspects of it you would change to strengthen its methodology?

References

Beard, L. B., & Johnson, A. T. (2024). Mapping psychological safety in the nursing classroom. *Teaching and Learning in Nursing*, *19*(2), 157–163. https://doi.org/10.1016/j.teln.2024.02.019

Blumer, H. (1969). *Symbolic interactionism: Perspective and method*. University of California Press.

Charmaz, K. (2014). *Constructing grounded theory* (2nd ed.). Sage.

Clarke, A. E. (2005). *Situational analysis: Grounded theory after the postmodern turn*. Sage.

Clarke, A. E. (2021). From grounded theory to situational analysis. What's new? Why? How? In J. M. Morse, B. J. Bowers, K. Charmaz, A. E. Clarke, J. Corbin, & C. J. Porr with P. N. Stern (Eds.), *Developing grounded theory: The second generation revisited* (pp. 223–266). Routledge.

Clarke, A. E., Friese, C., & Washburn, R. (2018). *Situational analysis: Grounded theory after the interpretive turn* (2nd ed.). Sage.

Foucault, M. (1973). *The order of things: An archeology of the human sciences*. Vintage Books.

Glaser, B. G. (1978). *Theoretical sensitivity: Advances in the methodology of grounded theory*. Sociology Press.

Glaser, B. G., & Strauss, A. (1967). *The discovery of grounded theory: Strategies for qualitative research*. Aldine de Gruyter.

Öhman, A., Keisu, B. I., & Enberg, B. (2023). Professional knowledge development and evidence-based practice in confusing vs. supportive work organizations: A grounded theory situational analysis of Swedish elderly care. *Physiotherapy Theory and Practice*, *39*(5), 994–1006. https://doi.org/10.1080/09593985.2022.2033370

Strauss, A. L. (1987). *Qualitative analysis for social scientists*. Cambridge University Press.

Strauss, A., & Corbin, J. (1990). *Basics of qualitative research: Techniques and procedures for developing grounded theory*. Sage.

Strauss, A., & Corbin, J. (1998). *Basics of qualitative research: Techniques and procedures for developing grounded theory* (2nd ed.). Sage.

Wiesner, K., Hein, K., Borasio, G. D., & Führer, M. (2024). "Collateral beauty". Experiences and needs of professionals caring for parents continuing pregnancy after a life-limiting prenatal diagnosis: A grounded theory study. *Palliative Medicine*, *38*(6), 679–688. https://doi.org/10.1177/02692163241255509

7

KATHY CHARMAZ'S CONSTRUCTIVIST GROUNDED THEORY

Charmaz was a member of the first cohort of PhD students in sociology at University of California San Francisco (UCSF). In the preface of her first edition of *Constructing Grounded Theory: A Practical Guide through Qualitative Analysis*, Charmaz (2006) shared she had the privilege of learning grounded theory from Glaser. She had enrolled in multiple graduate seminars he taught. Strauss was her dissertation chair. She explained that both Glaser and Strauss' influence permeated her work as she became a second-generation grounded theorist. Charmaz (2006; 2009) carefully decided on the name for her second-generation grounded theory. She chose "constructivist" to highlight subjectivity and the researcher's active involvement in constructing and interpreting data. In Charmaz's method emphasis is placed on flexible guidelines. Unlike Glaser and Strauss (1967) focus on discovering theory that emerged from data that are separate from the researcher, Charmaz's position is neither data nor theory are discovered as given in the data. Instead Charmaz emphasized that researchers are part of the world they study, the data they collect, and their analysis. Researchers construct grounded theory studies by means of their past and current interactions with individuals and research practices. Researchers are not separate from what they study but instead are a part of it. Charmaz published three editions of her *Constructing Grounded Theory* book (2006; 2014; 2025). After her death, the third edition was published in 2025.

Charmaz (2021) also found Corbin and Strauss' (2015) grounded theory approach to be too prescriptive with its paradigm matrix and coding. In constructivist grounded theory, Charmaz developed her version to separate it from the positivists' elements in Glaserian and Corbin and Strauss' grounded theory. Pragmatism instead of positivism provided the epistemological

DOI: 10.4324/9781032695563-7

underpinning of constructivist grounded theory. Pragmatism views our reality as fluid where there are multiple perspectives, and it has a problem-solving approach.

Charmaz (2021) argued that researchers' positionality is crucial. Researchers need to engage in strong reflexivity so they can develop what she calls "methodological self-consciousness" (p. 161) where researchers become aware of the privileges they take for granted. As pragmatists attend to social reform and solutions to practical problems, Charmaz's (2017) constructivist grounded theory was easily linked with critical inquiry which addresses power, inequality, and injustice. Charmaz (2021) declared that:

> We not only must excavate the preconceptions inherent in our worldviews but must examine our taken-for-granted privileges embedded in our various positions. Wealth, status, race, gender, age, and professional and other affiliations can shape our views of our research participants, their worlds, and our interpretations of them.
>
> *(p. 160)*

Researchers' steps to develop their methodological self-consciousness help their critical stance emerge and change how researchers view their participants, their research goals, and themselves. Researchers can scrutinize their privileges and priorities and how they impact their research process and relationships with their participants. Data can help researchers look beneath and beyond their privileges to help change their views. Charmaz and Belgrave (2019) emphasized how researchers regard data and analyze them are dependent on which version of grounded theory they adopt. Glaser (2013) stressed no preconceptions in his grounded theory methodology, but Charmaz emphasized that when researchers go deeper into their preconceptions, they can find obstacles that hinder developing critical inquiry.

Charmaz's (2025) constructivist grounded theory does share some methodological strategies of other versions of grounded theory. These common research practices include (1) constant comparative method of going back and forth between collecting and analyzing data, (2) creating inductive conceptual categories through coding, (3) memoing, and (4) developing a new theory instead of relying on applying existing theories.

Constructivist grounded theory has a renewed interest in studying process. Interviews are viewed as emergent interactions and can lead in unanticipated directions. Language and meaning are the focus. The bones of constructivist grounded theory, as in other grounded theory versions, are generating coding to provide a working skeleton. Charmaz's (2025) version involved two main phases. The first phase is initial coding which involves naming each word, line, or segment of data. The second phase is focused coding where the most significant initial codes are organized and integrated.

In initial coding Charmaz asks similar questions that Glaser (1978) did: "What is this data a study of?" (p. 57). When doing initial coding, the analyst needs to stay close to the data. Initial codes should be short and simple. Attempt to code for actions. Sensitizing concepts from symbolic interactionism can help in this first phase of coding. Codes at this stage are provisional and give researchers ideas to pursue in subsequent data collection.

During focused coding, researchers make decisions on which initial codes need to be categorized and condensed and highlight what the researchers decide as important in the emerging analysis. Focus codes are more conceptual than initial codes and have greater analytic power. Charmaz (2025) explained that her coding is different from Corbin and Strauss' axial coding because her analytic strategies are emergent and not procedural. In Glaser' (1978) grounded theory, theoretical coding has a place of prominence to help theorize data and help know how substantive code are related. Charmaz (2025) included a word of caution about theoretical codes because they may "lend an aura of objectivity to an analysis" (p. 156). Her advice was "If you use theoretical codes, let them break through the analysis, not be applied to it" (p. 157).

KEY POINTS IN CHARMAZ'S CONSTRUCTIVIST GROUNDED THEORY

- Researchers co-construct grounded theory studies by means of their past and current interactions with participants.
- Researchers are not separate from what they investigate but rather are a part of it.
- Researchers' positionality is crucial; they need to engage in strong reflexivity so they can develop "methodological self-consciousness".
- Constructivist grounded theory is linked with critical inquiry which focuses on power, inequality, and injustice.
- Two main phases of coding include initial coding and focused coding.

Theoretical sensitivity will help researchers bring analytic precision to their analysis. Charmaz sees theoretical sensitivity and codes influencing each other. Theoretical sensitivity refers to the researcher's ability to understand data in abstract terms to identify abstract relationships among their constructive categories. For Charmaz (2025) memo writing is the critical step between collecting data and analyzing the data. In memo writing researchers stop to analyze an idea about their codes and increase the level of abstraction of their focused codes to conceptual categories.

TABLE 7.1 Progression of Charmaz's Constructivist Grounded Theory Publications

2006	Constructing Grounded Theory: A Practical Guide through Qualitative Analysis
2009	Shifting the Grounds: Constructivist Grounded Theory Methods in Morse et al. Developing Grounded Theory: The Second Generation
2014	Constructing Grounded Theory (2nd Edition)
2021	The Genesis, Grounds, and Growth of Constructivist Grounded Theory in Morse et al. Developing Grounded Theory: The Second Generation Revisited
2025	Constructing Grounded Theory (3rd Edition)

Theoretical sampling is the strategy used to seek and collect additional data to refine properties of categories in a developing grounded theory. Theoretical sampling involves abduction which is a form of reasoning when researchers cannot account for puzzling or unexpected findings. Here researchers go back and forth between data and their theoretical category to explain the puzzling findings. Theoretical sampling helps to identify gaps among categories and discover variation within a category or process.

In Charmaz's grounded theory, memos, sorting, and diagrams are interrelated processes in the theoretical development of researchers' analysis. Sorting the written analytic memos, comparing them, and integrating them help create and refine theoretical links in the merging theory. Charmaz suggested turning off the computer and sorting memos by hand on a large table where you can see them and rearrange them. Diagramming the emerging grounded theory provides a visual representation of categories and their relationships. Diagrams give an emerging theory an analytic frame where researchers can more easily see if any revisions are needed to the theory.

In coding and memoing Charmaz stressed using gerunds like Glaser and Strauss (1967) advocated. Gerunds encourage thinking about actions and analyzing actions. Charmaz called for emphasis on actions and processes as a critical strategy in constructing theory rather than categorizing individuals as the unit of analysis. Studying process helps construct a theory because it helps researchers conceptualize relationships between experiences and events and define major phases in the process. Charmaz warned that a hazard in grounded theory is making a list of connected but under analyzed processes.

The progression of her publications is provided in Table 7.1.

Interdisciplinary Examples of Constructivist Grounded Theory

The discipline of business was represented by this constructivist grounded theory study in Finland. Hytti et al. (2024) examined how fatherhood shaped entrepreneurial masculinities in the Finnish context where there are strong gender equality norms. The investigation focused on how father entrepreneurs enacted entrepreneurial masculinities while maintaining the intersection of work and family life. Using theoretical sampling, Hytti et al. focused on selecting funders of technology ventures. Twenty-two life stories were collected as directed by Charmaz and Belgrave (2012). Using Charmaz's constructivist grounded theory approach, Hytti et al. discovered that entrepreneurial masculinities were rooted in hegemonic masculinity either openly or subtly. How men maintained unequal gender relations with their spouses or other men were present in all the participants' accounts. The three main mechanisms to achieve this were (1) downplaying fatherhood to justify heroic entrepreneurial masculinity, (2) enacting ceremonial fatherhood to celebrate entrepreneurial breadwinner masculinity, and (3) claiming fatherhood as pivotal to rationalizing entrepreneurial caring masculinity.

In a focus on higher education in Norway, Ristad et al. (2024) conducted a constructivist grounded theory study to investigate the decision-making process that leads professionals to either take or not to take actions regarding inclusion of students with disabilities in higher education. Data were collected from 6 workshops with 46 multiple stakeholders such as students with disabilities, faculty, and support personnel. Initial coding of transcripts from workshops using gerunds was followed by focus coding. Researchers wrote analytic memos throughout the analysis and constructed the professionals' decision-making process. There were three phases, stakeholders explained, that influenced their decision to act or not. The first was exposing a weak individual foundation of knowledge and skills to perform their duties effectively for students with disabilities. The next phase involved exposing cracks in the university system. Stakeholders emphasized the need for mandatory inclusion training and creating a culture of inherent inclusion. The last phase in the decision-making process of making the final call on inclusion of students with disabilities was ruling based on knowledge and attitudes.

In Italy Baldi et al. (2024) from the discipline of medicine conducted a constructivist grounded theory study of gastric cancer patients returning to eating after a total gastrectomy. Their research question was "What is the process of returning to eating and feeding after a gastrectomy?" (p. 2). Semi-structured interviews were performed with 11 gastric cancer patients, 2 caregivers, and 5 physicians for a total sample of 18 participants. The analysis included open, focus, and theoretical coding. During focus coding, 15 provisional categories were identified. Next the researchers used theoretical sampling in their constant comparison and interviewed four additional gastric cancer patients to saturate categories. During theoretical coding, categories decreased in number. The process discovered, which was the core category, was defining a balance by compromising with fear. These fears were of becoming sick by eating and of a tumor recurrence. The process consisted of four main phases: Relying on the doctor's advice, perceptive realignment, rearranging food intake, and food-regulated social interactions.

In the discipline of psychology using Charmaz's constructivist grounded theory approach, Hinger et al. (2023) investigated racial allyship from the perspective of Black, Indigenous, and People of Color (BIPOC). Racial allyship referred to White persons working to end racism and white supremacy. The majority of racial allyship research has been from the perspective of White allies. Hinger et al.'s research question was "How do BIPOC define racial allyship in their own lives?" (p. 632). Their study was informed by critical race theory. Twenty-nine college BIPOC undergraduate students in eight focus group sessions comprised the sample. Hinger et al. incorporated reflexivity and positionality, which are the key components of constructivist grounded theory. In fact, they included a table that identified the positionality of all ten authors. The table consisted of the following columns for each author: (1) Salient identities, (2) key biases, assumptions, and areas of less awareness, and (3) strategies used to account for key biases, assumptions, and diminished awareness. After open coding, researchers engaged in focused coding and then theoretical coding. The core category of committing fully to allyship included six categories: Building trust, engaging in action, critical awareness, sociopolitical knowledge, accountability, and communicating/disseminating information. Findings have implications for White counseling psychologists helping them to incorporate racial allyship to promote social justice, multiculturalism, and prevention.

In the discipline of Social Work comes a constructivist grounded theory study on transmasculine self-defense and collective protection at clinical settings (Jordan, 2024). This grounded theory focused on how transgender persons negotiate their care and challenging patterns of marginalization and exclusion in clinical settings. Jordan's choice of a constructivist grounded theory approach aligned perfectly with Charmaz's social justice lens in helping to rectify inequities in health care systems. Based on Charmaz's emphasis on researcher reflexivity, Jordan included his researcher positionality. "I am a White transmasculine person and longtime participant in social movements for trans liberation and racial and economic justice" (p. 2). Jordan defined "transmasculine" broadly as "assigned female at birth and currently identifying as: a man, male, transgender, two spirit, non-binary or gender nonconforming" (p. 2). Jordan interviewed 26 transmasculine persons using videoconferencing and used reflexive analysis to interrogate his experiences of navigating health care. Jordan used line-by-line open coding with analytic memos to identify focused codes. Theoretical sampling helped expand emergent analyses. The reflexive memos helped this researcher engage with emotions and preconceived ideas and separate these from interpretations during data analysis. Compelling care, the actions and feelings that went into making healthcare experiences different, was the central theoretical focus. In this grounded theory compelling care explained how participants gained agency over their care through daily acts to defend themselves. The processes involved in compelling care included preparing for a fight, vetting providers, refusing biomedical gender categorization, directing treatment, and pursuing accountability.

In Germany Eckardt and Dorsch (2025) from the field of sports and exercise conducted a constructivist grounded theory of cooperation among parents, coaches, and administrators in professional youth soccer academies. The sample consisted of 9 parents, 11 coaches, and 14 administrators who were interviewed via online videoconferencing. Guided by Charmaz's method, data were analyzed using both initial and focused coding and theoretical integration. The resulting grounded theory included three processes of building, maintaining, and reinforcing cooperation. In building cooperation parents became familiar with the academy and navigated involvement. Interpersonal actions that parents, coaches, and administrators used to maintain cooperation were the focus of the second process. Reinforcing cooperation involved a dynamic, responsive, and iterative process which included a feedback culture that helped sustain the operations of academies.

End-of-Chapter Student Exercise

For this exercise focus your search on your own discipline be it psychology, education, nursing, business, social work, etc. Search for the past 5 years the database used most frequently in your discipline to locate constructivist grounded theory studies. Select one study and use the following guide questions to comment on its methodology:

1 Did the researchers follow Charmaz's constructivist grounded theory methodology? If not, which aspects of her approach were not followed?
2 Did the researchers identify the epistemological underpinning of their study?
3 Did the researchers address their positionality and how they practiced reflexivity while conducting their constructivist grounded theory study?
4 Were Charmaz's two main phases of coding used? Initial coding and focused coding?
5 Did the researchers identify a process central to their findings?
6 Did the topic of the study focus on power, inequality, and injustice? If yes, what specific topic did the researchers study to help remedy the situation?
7 If you were to conduct this study using Charmaz's constructivist grounded theory approach, are there any aspects of it you would revise to strengthen its methodology?

References

Baldi, L., D'Incá, M., Wildner, J., Tecce, F., DePasco, R., Finotto, S., Crescitelli, M. E. D., DiLeo, S., & Ghirotto, L. (2024). Defining a balance by compromising with fear: A grounded theory study on returning to eating after a total gastrectomy. *Palliative and Supportive Care*. https://doi.org/10.1017/S1478951523002031

Charmaz, K. (2006). *Constructing grounded theory: A practical guide through qualitative analysis.* Sage.

Charmaz, K. (2009). Shifting grounds: Constructivist ground theory methods. In J. M. Morse, P. N. Stern, J. Corbin, B. Bowers, K. Charmaz, & A. E. Clarke (Eds.), *Developing grounded theory: The second generation.* Left Coast Press.

Charmaz, K. (2014). *Constructing grounded theory* (2nd ed.). Sage.

Charmaz, K. (2021). The genesis, grounds, and growth of constructivist grounded theory. In J. M. Morse, B. J. Bowers, K. Charmaz, A. E. Clarke, J. Corbin, & C. J. Porr with P. N. Stern (Eds.), *Developing grounded theory: The second generation revisited.* (pp. 153–187). Routledge.

Charmaz, K. (2025). *Constructing grounded theory* (3rd ed.). Sage.

Charmaz, K., & Belgrave, L. L. (2012), Qualitative interviewing and grounded theory analysis. In J. Gubrium, J. A. Holstein, A. B. Marvasti, & K. D. McKinneyet (Eds.), *The Sage handbook of interview research: The complexity of the craft* (pp. 347–366). Sage.

Charmaz, K., & Belgrave, L. L. (2019). Thinking about data with grounded theory. *Qualitative Inquiry, 25*(8), 743–753. https://doi.org/10.1177/1077800418809455

Corbin, J., & Strauss, A. (2015). *Basics of qualitative research: Techniques and procedures for developing grounded theory* (4th ed.). Sage.

Eckardt, V. C., & Dorsch, T. E. (2025). "We are on the outside but it's okay": A grounded theory of cooperation between parents, coaches, and administrators in professional youth soccer academies. *Psychology of Sport & Exercise, 76,* 102746. https://doi.org/10.1016/j.psychsport.2024.102746

Glaser, B. G. (1978). *Theoretical sensitivity: Advances in the methodology of grounded theory.* Sociology Press.

Glaser, B. G. (2013). *No preconceptions: The grounded theory dictum.* Sociology Press.

Glaser, B. G., & Strauss, A. (1967). *The discovery of grounded theory: Strategies for qualitative research.* Aldine de Gruyter.

Hinger, C. L., DeBlaere, C., Gwira, R., Aiello, M., Punjwani, A., Cobourne, L., Tran, N., Lord, M., Mike., J., & Green, C. (2023). Defining racial allies: A qualitative investigation of white allyship from the perspective of people of color. *Journal of Counseling Psychology, 70*(6), 631–644. https://doi.org/10.1037/cou0000709

Hytti, U., Karhunen, P., & Radu-Lefebvre, M. (2024). Entrepreneurial masculinity: A fatherhood perspective. *Entrepreneurship Theory and Practice, 48*(1), 246–273. https://doi.org/10.1177/10422587231155863

Jordan, S. P. (2024). Compelling care: A grounded theory of transmasculine self-defense and collective protection at the clinic. *Social Science and Medicine, 345,* 116638. https://doi.org/10.1016/j.socscimed.2024.116638

Ristad, T., Ostvik, J., Horghagen, S., Kvam, L., & Witso, A. E. (2024). A multi-stakeholder perspective on inclusion in higher education: Ruling on fragile ground. *International Journal of Educational Research Open, 6,* 100311. https://doi.org/10.1016/j.ijedro.2023.100311

8

COMPARISON OF FIRST- AND SECOND- GENERATION GROUNDED THEORY APPROACHES

Almost 60 years have passed since Glaser and Strauss (1967) first developed grounded theory. Some of their PhD students became the second generation of grounded theory methodologists. Juliet Corbin collaborated with Strauss and then continued to modify their grounded theory approach after Strauss' passing. Three other doctoral students Adele Clarke, Kathy Charmaz, and Barbara Bowers with one postdoctoral fellow, Leonard Schatzman, developed their own versions of grounded theory: Situational analysis, constructivist grounded theory, and dimensional analysis, respectively. Glaser's PhD students continued with his classic grounded theory and did not see the need to develop any new approaches. Physllis Noerager Stern (2013) worked closely with Glaser, and she wrote "I have kept to the processes of the original method because it works for me, it's systematic, and the products are applicable. I advise you to do the same" (p. 167). Stern (1994) was the first person to label the two versions of grounded theory as Glaserian and Straussian after each of the developers.

Researchers have so many choices when deciding on which grounded theory approach to use for their studies. Figure 8.1 shows a decisions tree that can help researchers decide which grounded theory approach fits best with their proposed research study. Table 8.1 shows a comparison among the five grounded theory approaches in terms of epistemological foundations, researcher's role, research questions, timing of literature review, and data analysis. Straussian grounded theory is divided into two columns in the table. First is Strauss and Corbin's 1990 and 1998 versions and then Corbin and Strauss' 2008 and 2015 versions of their approach.

As mentioned earlier in this book, one grounded theory approach is not better than another. It depends on the right match between the grounded

DOI: 10.4324/9781032695563-8

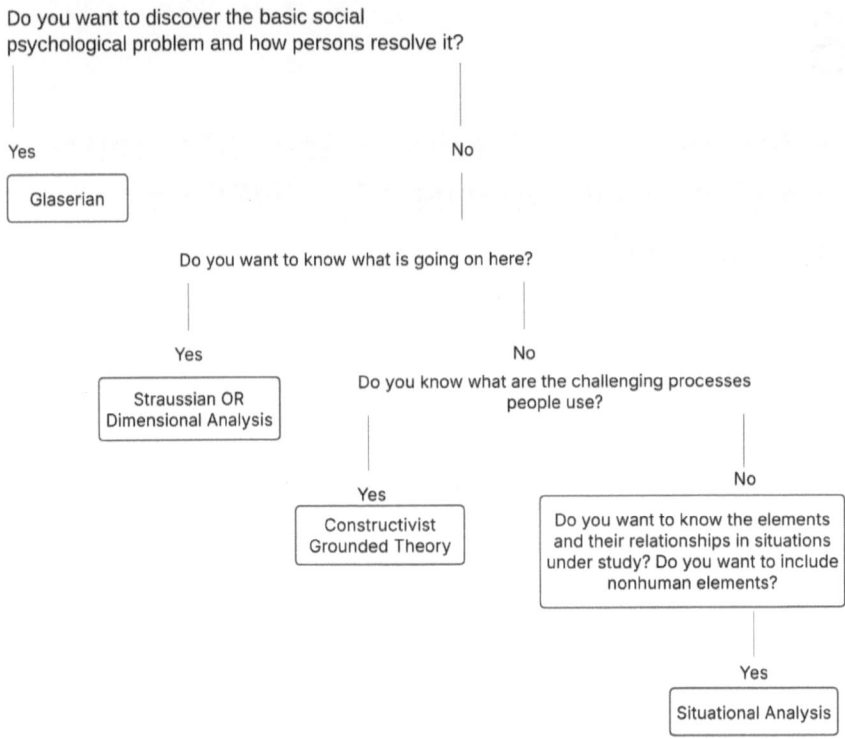

FIGURE 8.1   Decision Tree for Research Questions

theorist's philosophy, research question, researcher's role, the population under study, and the outcome desired. Does the researcher want to discover the
basic problem the participants experience and the process they use to cope
or resolve this problem? If so, Glaserian grounded theory would be a perfect
match. Researchers should remember that Glaser stressed the importance of
theoretical codes in grounded theory. He even published an entire book on
theoretical coding (Glaser, 2005).

  If instead the researcher wants to focus on the situation itself and not a
basic problem, then Clarke et al.'s (2018) situational analysis would be an
appropriate match. Clarke et al.'s method focuses on what elements are in
the situation under study and how they are related. If researchers prefer a
less rigid and more flexible approach to analysis, maybe Corbin and Strauss's
(2015) grounded theory approach will be their choice. In choosing this approach, it should be noted that even though Corbin and Strauss stressed their
grounded theory approach is free flowing. Their coding process, however, of
inserting data into the paradigm of conditions, interactions, and consequences is procedural. Bowers and Schatzman's (2021) dimensional analysis
also uses Strauss' matrix but as an overarching framework for the study.

TABLE 8.1 Comparisons of the Grounded Theory Approaches

Characteristic	Glaserian	Strauss and Corbin (1990; 1998)	Corbin and Strauss (2008; 2015)	Dimensional Analysis	Constructivist Grounded Theory	Situational Analysis
Epistemological foundations	Positivism Symbolic interaction	Positivism Pragmatism Symbolic interaction	Pragmatism Social interaction Feminism Constructivism	Symbolic interaction	Pragmatism	Pragmatism Social interaction Foucault's work Deleuze & Guattari's concepts of rhizome and assembling
Researcher's role	Neutral observer	Interaction between researcher, data, and participants	Co-constructed Sensitivity Self-reflection Social justice	Both perspectives of the researcher and the participants are essential in analysis	Co-constructed data and analysis with participants Reflexivity Critical social justice	Reflexivity Critical social justice
Research questions	What is the basic social psychological problem? What is the process people use to cope or resolve that problem?	What is going on here?	Frame question in a way that provides flexibility to explore topic being studied	What all is involved here?	What are the challenging situations and processes people use?	What are the elements and their relations in a situation under study?

(Continued)

TABLE 8.1 (Continued)

Characteristic	Glaserian	Strauss and Corbin (1990; 1998)	Corbin and Strauss (2008; 2015)	Dimensional Analysis	Constructivist Grounded Theory	Situational Analysis
Prior literature review	No	Yes	Yes	Yes	Yes	Yes
Data analysis	Substantive coding • Open • Selective Theoretical coding	Open coding Axial coding Selective coding Conditional/ consequential Matrix • Conditions • Actions and interactions • Consequences/ outcomes	Open coding Axial coding Selective coding Updated diagram of conditional/ consequential matrix	Exploratory matrix • Context • Conditions • Processes • Consequences	Initial coding Focused coding	Four kinds of maps • Situational • Relational • Social worlds/ arenas • Positional

Clarke et al.'s (2018) grounded theory approach is the only approach that does not use coding. Clarke et al.'s four maps are central to data analysis where the situation under study is the unit of analysis, which does not involve coding. Clarke et al.'s situational analysis is the only grounded theory approach that includes non-human entities. Clarke's analysis is a very different type of analysis. Their maps are not conceptual and do not include analytic diagrams based on grounded theory codes.

If critical social justice and healthcare disparities are the researcher's interests, then Charmaz's constructivist grounded theory will be a perfect choice. Her method concentrates on identifying processes. Charmaz (2025) noted a word of caution about theoretical codes in her approach because she felt they may provide an impression of objectivity to the analysis. Even though Charmaz's approach focuses on investigating social justice issues, it does not mean that a grounded theorist is prevented from studying all these important issues using any of the other approaches.

Researchers' positionality and reflexivity are important components to consider in choosing a grounded theory approach. In Bowers and Schatzman's (2021) dimensional analysis, both perspectives of the researcher and the participants are essential in the analysis. They explained that when researchers do not take their perspectives into account during data analysis, there is a possibility they can misinterpret the data. In their situational analysis, Clarke et al. (2018) urged that intentional reflexivity is an essential part of the research process. Charmaz (2025) brought the most attention to grounded theorists analyzing data together with their participants by calling her approach, constructivist grounded theory. This brought researchers' reflexivity front and center in her approach. Strauss and Corbin (1990; 1998) in their first editions of their approach did not address reflexivity. In later editions, however, Corbin and Strauss (2008; 2015) did begin to address reflexivity and co-construction of grounded theory with participants as Corbin included feminism and constructivism in these editions. Classic Glaserian grounded theory does not address reflexivity or co-construction of analysis. There is nothing, however, to prevent grounded theorists using the Glaserian approach to frame their study with a constructivist epistemological foundation instead of positivism where researchers can co-construct the findings with their participants.

In only Glaser's classic grounded theory approach, researchers are urged not to delve too deeply into reviewing the literature prior to starting their studies. I have used classic grounded theory in my two studies I have presented in this book. I did review the literature but not in depth prior to starting both my studies. I feel that researchers do need to know what research has already been conducted on the topic they are proposing to study. Also being in a practice discipline of nursing, as a clinician I wanted to be up to date on research on the topic I was studying, postpartum depression, in case my participants had any questions about this postpartum mood disorder they were experiencing. I felt it was the least I could do for them in return for participating in my studies.

References

Bowers, B. J., & Schatzman, L. (2021). Dimensional analysis. In J. M. Morse, B. J. Bowers, K. Charmaz, A. E. Clarke, J. Corbin, C. Porr, & with P. N. Stern (Eds.), *Developing grounded theory: The second generation revisited* (pp. 111–129). Routledge.

Charmaz, K. (2025). *Constructing grounded theory* (3rd ed.). Sage.

Clarke, A. E., Friese, C., & Washburn, R. S. (2018). *Situational analysis: Grounded theory after the interpretive turn.* Sage.

Corbin, J., & Strauss, A. (2008). *Basics of qualitative research: Techniques and procedures for developing grounded theory* (3rd ed.). Sage.

Corbin, J., & Strauss, A. (2015). *Basics of qualitative research: Techniques and procedures for developing grounded theory* (4th ed.). Sage.

Glaser, B. G. (2005). *The grounded theory perspective III: Theoretical coding.* Sociology Press.

Glaser, B. G., & Strauss, L. (1967). *The discovery of grounded theory: Strategies for qualitative research.* Aldine de Gruyter.

Stern, P. N. (1994). Eroding grounded theory, In J. Morse (Ed.), *Critical issues in qualitative inquiry* (pp. 212–223). Sage.

Stern, P. N. (2013). Glaserian grounded theory" the enduring method. In C. T. Beck (Ed.), *Routledge international handbook of qualitative nursing research* (pp. 162–168). Routledge.

Strauss, A., & Corbin, J. (1990). *Basics of qualitative research: Techniques and procedures for developing grounded theory.* Sage.

Strauss, A., & Corbin, J. (1998). *Basics of qualitative research: Techniques and procedures for developing grounded theory* (2nd ed.). Sage.

9

CRITIQUING GROUNDED THEORY STUDIES

In this chapter criteria for evaluating grounded theory research offered by different grounded theorists are included. The checklists of Birk and Mills (2023), Charmaz (2006; 2014), Corbin and Strauss (2008), Glaser (1978), Glaser and Strauss (1967), Schatzman and Strauss (1973), and Strauss and Corbin (1990; 1998) are described. The criteria for assessing different grounded theory approaches offered by Morse et al. (2021) in their book, *Developing Grounded Theory: The Second Generation* are also addressed in this chapter. Many of the criteria of these grounded theorists overlap and some focus on different aspects of a grounded theory's methodology used.

Glaser and Strauss' Criteria

Glaser and Strauss (1967) gave advice for judging the credibility of a grounded theory study. A reader's judgment on the credibility will be based on their assessment of the variety of events the researchers included: Who they interviewed, what different groups were compared, and what types of data were utilized. Multiple comparison groups increase the credibility of a theory. Glaser and Strauss called for analysts to describe their data of the social world they collected in order for the readers to almost see and hear the participants in relation to the grounded theory being developed. Another suggestion for increasing credibility was to include a description of the procedures used to analyze the data.

Glaser and Strauss (1967) also provided criteria for evaluating the practical application of a grounded theory study. To apply a grounded theory, there are at least four interrelated properties: Fit, understanding, generality, and control. Fit refers to the theory fitting in the substantive area where it will be used. A grounded theory needs to be sufficiently general so that it can be applied to

DOI: 10.4324/9781032695563-9

many diverse situations in the substantive area. A grounded theory needs to make sense and be understandable by people concerned with the topic of study. The conceptual levels of categories in a grounded theory need to be general enough to allow the theory flexibility enough to guide multiple conditional and constantly changing situations. Lastly regarding the property of control, when persons apply a theory, they need to be able to understand ongoing situations, predict change in them, and control consequences. Glaser and Strauss explained that "the crux of controllability is the production and control of change though 'controllable' variables and access variables." (Glaser & Strauss, 1967, p. 245).

Glaser's Criteria

Glaser (1978) updated his criteria for application of a grounded theory. For fit, the categories of the theory need to fit the data collected and fit the realities under study. Glaser used the term work to refer to the theory being able to explain what occurred, predict what will happen, and interpret what is occurring in the substantive area. A grounded theory works if it can explain the main variations in behavior in the substantive area being studied in regard to processing the basic problem of participants. The theory next needs to be relevant to the action in the substantive area. In grounded theory relevance is achieved because it permits core problems and processes to emerge from data and not come from preconceived theories. Lastly modifiability is an important criterion because generation of a grounded theory is an ever-changing process. The theory should not be written in stone so that it can be modified when new data are collected. In 1992 Glaser added two more criteria, those being, parsimony and scope in explanatory power.

Morse et al., (2021, pp. 302–304) listed the following strategies for strong Glaserian grounded theory research:

- Focus consistently on moving data analysis to an abstract explanatory level.
- Use constant comparative method of analysis.
- Always use theoretical sampling.
- Appropriately measure rigor of the methods.
- Relevance.
- Modifiability.

Schatzman and Strauss' Criteria

In their 1973 book, *Field Research: Strategies for a Natural Sociology*, Schatzman and Strauss concentrated on how to establish credibility. A critical prerequisite to establish credibility is the researchers' conviction that what they are writing is in fact so. This conviction is based on the credible procedures the researchers performed. Schatzman and Strauss explained that for every proposition, data are empirically and logically related to the proposition. Host verification is another aspect of credibility that addresses if major propositions are checked by experiences of hosts. There are two questions they offered to assess this. "Would an independent observer make conceptual discoveries that empirically or logically invalidate his own? Would another social science analyst, examining only the actual raw data reach the same conclusions?" (Schatzman & Strauss, 1973, p. 134). Phenomenon recognition is another criterion for establishing credibility. It examines whether other people who are knowledgeable about the phenomenon under study, either by researching it or experiencing it themselves, recognize the phenomenon in the analysis. Schatzman and Strauss offered this question to help assess this criterion: "Does the researcher's analysis, which was probably based upon a different perspective or framework from theirs, actually help the audience explain-albeit in a new way- their own experiences?" (p. 135).

Strauss and Corbin's Criteria

Strauss and Corbin's (1990, pp. 254–256) first set of criteria regarding empirical grounding of a theory included:

- Are concepts identified?
- Are the concepts systematically related?
- Do categories have conceptual density?
- Are there linkages among the categories?
- Is variation evident in the theory?
- Has analysis focused on process?
- Do the results seem significant?

In the second edition of Strauss and Corbin's (1998) book, they added one more criterion: "Does the theory stand the test of time and become part of the discussions and ideas exchanged among relevant social and professional groups?" (p. 272).

Corbin and Strauss (2008) added more criteria for judging the quality of research using grounded theory method. The first criterion is fit; the second is applicability or usefulness of the results. The third criterion focuses on concepts and the development of their properties and dimensions. The fourth criterion is the contextualization of concepts. Results need to be described in relation to their context. Logic is the fifth criterion where one looks if there is a logical flow of ideas in the theory. The depth of findings is concentrated in the sixth criterion. Richness and details in the results are necessary. The seventh criterion focuses on variation being built into the findings to demonstrate complexity. Creativity is the eighth criterion which concentrates on how findings are creatively presented. Sensitivity to the participants and data is the ninth criterion. The final criterion refers to evidence of memo writing.

Corbin and Strauss (2015) disliked using the word "criteria" because that implies an all or nothing view of evaluation. Instead, they now prefer the term "checkpoints". They created a list of checkpoints for evaluating the methodological consistency of a grounded theory study and a list of checkpoints for evaluating the quality and applicability of a grounded theory study. Examples of some of their checkpoints are included here. To evaluate methodological consistency of a grounded theory study, some of their checkpoints include:

- Was theoretical sampling used?
- How were data collected?
- Was constant comparison of data done?
- Were any examples of memos included?
- Did the grounded theorists describe their coding process?
- Did the grounded theorists describe their methodological decisions?
- Did the grounded theorists keep a research journal?
- Were ethical considerations addressed?
- Did the researchers obtain feedback from the participants and/or other professionals?

Next to evaluate the quality and applicability of a grounded theory study, Corbin and Strauss' (2015) checklist include the following checkpoints:

- Did the researchers identify the core category and how the categories related to it?
- Were the context, conditions, and consequences integrated into the theory?
- Did the researchers explain how saturation was achieved?
- Did the results resonate with professionals' experiences?
- Do the results appear significant?
- Did researchers provide implications for practice, policy, and teaching based on their results?

Morse et al. (2021) identified these criteria to assess Straussian grounded theory research: Goodness of fit, applicability of results, concepts, conceptualization of concepts, logic, depth, variation, creativity, sensitivity, and evidence of memoing.

Charmaz's Criteria

Charmaz (2006; 2014; 2025) argued that whoever the audience is, they will judge the usefulness of the grounded theory methods by the quality of the final product. Charmaz included four main criteria for evaluating grounded theory:

Credibility, originality, resonance, and usefulness. She explained that a strong combination of the first two criteria, credibility and originality, increases the other criteria of resonance and usefulness. These four criteria focus on the empirical study and how the theory was developed. As Charmaz pointed out, her criteria do not evaluate the esthetics of the researcher's writing on the grounded theory study. Credibility focuses on how sufficient are the data that the researchers based the grounded theory on and how strong are the theoretical links between the data and analysis. Originality examines if the grounded theory study revealed any new insights or concepts. When assessing resonance, an evaluator looks at whether the grounded theory results make sense to the sample participants and to other persons who share their same circumstances. Usefulness encompasses whether the grounded theory findings can be used in everyday life and if they contribute to knowledge to help improve persons' lives. Can the results lead to future research in other substantive topics?

Morse et al. (2021) included the following criteria for strong constructivist grounded theory research:

- Assume multiple realities among participants and the grounded theorists.
- Assume mutual construction of findings through interaction between researchers and participants.
- Assume that the grounded theorists themselves construct categories of analysis.
- Assume that the observers' values, priorities, positions, and actions impact their views.
- View generalizations only as partial and conditional based in time, space, positions, and interaction. Do not overgeneralize.
- Identify the range of variations within the dataset and in the possible interpretations of that dataset.
- Strive to develop a theory that is credible and original, has resonance, and is useful.
- View co-constructed data at the start of analysis rather at the end of the analytic process.
- Strive to engage in reflexivity throughout the research process and reflect on the impact of your positionality on your interpretation.

Situational Analysis

Morse et al. (2021) addressed the following criteria for strong situational analysis:

- Is the grounded theory situated-located in space, time, and history in written memos?
- Are all the key components involved in the situation completely analyzed in situational maps and memos?

- Are the key relations among the elements fully analyzed in relational maps and memos?
- Are the specifics of the broader situation included in social worlds/arena maps and memos?
- Have all the important collective entities in the situation and their commitments been analyzed?
- Have all the main debates in the discourse materials located in the situation been analyzed in positional maps and memos?
- Were nonhuman elements in the situation identified and their consequences for others in the situation analyzed and memoed?

Dimensional Analysis

The following criteria were identified by Morse et al. (2021) for strong dimensional analysis research:

- Have clarity regarding the perspectives of various sources of data.
- Include relevant perspectives in data analysis.
- Explain the implications of power differences of varying perspectives.
- Identify how perspectives in literature are similar or different from perspectives found in data sources in the study.
- Be guided by symbolic interaction with a focus on process during analysis.
- Develop conceptual matrices during data analysis.
- Identify dimensions found in the different data sources and their relationships to perspective.
- Use of interview questions that help identify relevant dimensions and their relationships with each other.
- Avoid bringing the researcher's own categories to the data analysis.
- Identify conditions related to differences in dimensions and their configurations.

Birk and Mills (2023) also have three criteria for evaluating grounded theory research. These criteria are researcher expertise, methodological congruence, and procedural precision. Some aspects of the researchers' expertise that can be assessed focus on their scholarly writing skills and familiarity with grounded theory methods. For the criterion of methodological congruence, Birk and Mills suggest looking at whether the researchers stated their philosophical position, if grounded theory was the appropriate method to match their purpose of the study, and was a grounded theory presented as the outcome of the study? Procedural precision is the third main criterion and involves assessing if the researchers showed evidence of memoing, an audit trail, procedures for data management, logical connections between the data and their abstractions, and are applications of their results identified?

References

Birk, M., & Mills, J. (2023). *Grounded theory: A practical guide*. Sage.

Charmaz, K. (2006). *Constructing grounded theory: A practical guide through qualitative analysis*. Sage.

Charmaz, K. (2014). *Constructing grounded theory* (2nd ed.). Sage.

Charmaz, K. (2025). *Constructing grounded theory* (3rd ed.). Sage.

Corbin, J., & Strauss, A. (2008). *Basics of qualitative research: Techniques and procedures for developing grounded theory* (3rd ed.). Sage.

Corbin, J., & Strauss, A. (2015). *Basics of qualitative research: Techniques and procedures for developing grounded theory* (4th ed.). Sage.

Glaser, B. G. (1978). *Theoretical sensitivity: Advances in the methodology of grounded theory*. Sociology Press.

Glaser, B. G. (1992). *Basics of grounded theory analysis: Emergence vs forcing*. Sociology Press.

Glaser, B. G., & Strauss, A. (1967). *The discovery of grounded theory: Strategies for qualitative research*. Aldine de Gruyter.

Morse, J. M., Bowers, B. J., Charmaz, K., Clarke, A. E., Corbin, J., & Porr, C. J. (Eds.). (2021). *Developing grounded theory: The second generation revisited*. Routledge.

Schatzman, L., & Strauss, A. L. (1973). *Field research: Strategies for a natural sociology*. Prentice-Hall, Inc.

Strauss, A., & Corbin, J. (1990). *Basics of qualitative research: Techniques and procedures for developing grounded theory*. Sage.

Strauss, A., & Corbin, J. (1998). *Basics of qualitative research: Techniques and procedures for developing grounded theory* (2nd ed.). Sage.

10

TEACHING GROUNDED THEORY

To help prepare our next generation of grounded theorists, teaching strategies take center stage in this chapter. First teaching approaches of Glaser and Charmaz are described. Next teaching approaches that other faculty have published are presented. Lastly I presented examples from my own teaching assignments that I use in my PhD courses at University of Connecticut School of Nursing.

Glaser's Teaching Strategies

Glaser (1998) presented several exercises that can help researchers learn grounded theory methodology to help improve and sharpen and also prevent poor techniques found in literature. The first exercise he called the five properties and can occur in a classroom setting. This exercise can help students get a feel for coding and category generation. Students are asked to decide on an experience that all the students in the class know and think of five properties of a possible core category. Class analysis is another exercise Glaser offered as a possibility for a class to be involved with over a series of classes. He called it a "doing" exercise. First the class decides on a topic they all know well. Each student in the class then shares an experience they had on that topic. Students compare each student's experience to the other one. Glaser suggested one student be designated as a memo recorder to take notes on the emerging categories and their properties. Another student can be chosen to record methodological occurrence on how the analysis is progressing. Students who wrote memos bring memos to the next class and then the classmates can start to sort them. This "doing" exercise goes for two to

DOI: 10.4324/9781032695563-10

three classes, so all students get the experience of going through the grounded theory process.

A grounded theory seminar is another possibility an experienced faculty member can offer as a semester long course (Glaser, 1998). Over the semester each student works on their own grounded theory project. During the classes students present the progress they are making on their projects and get feedback from their fellow classmates. The class gives each student feedback four times: Open coding, selective coding, memo sorting, and reworking the writing up of their papers. Glaser suggested there is a division of labor in the seminar: Positions for a presenter, two note takers, and then the analysts who are the remaining students in the class.

In Glaser's (2016) book, *The Cry for Help: Preserving Autonomy Doing GT Research*, he began the book with this stating:

> One of the precious properties of classical grounded theory is the autonomy it gives the researcher. A response to a cry for help from a novice ground theory researcher can take away his autonomy. It can be a strong answer by a strong senior researcher that undermines the emerging theory of the novice. The novice must be careful not to yield or give away his power of autonomy for a need for help, as desperate as he may feel the need.
>
> *(p. 1)*

Faculty supervising PhD students in their grounded theory dissertations must be patient as the novice researcher struggles to achieve comfort and confidence with the grounded theory methodology. Faculty can help their PhD students tolerate confusion as they begin their grounded theory dissertation. In supervising PhD students in their grounded theory dissertations, faculty who are experienced in grounded theory need to be careful that they do not take away their students' autonomy. A difficulty in researchers learning classic grounded theory is what Stern (1994) labeled as minus mentoring. Glaser explained that this occurs when researchers are trying to conduct grounded theory but there is no available mentor who is experienced in grounded theory available to them.

Charmaz's Teaching Exercises

Charmaz (2015) reflected on her teaching grounded theory. Overall, she called for a supportive environment which includes demonstrations, collective participation, specific tasks, and progressive analysis. There are three key areas of qualitative inquiry regarding grounded theory construction: Intensive interviewing, coding, and memo writing. Students in the class conduct a small empirical study, one that can be completed in a semester. They collect and analyze qualitative interview data. They critique their interview guide and correct some weak questions in their guide. To help students learn coding, Charmaz has students engage in line-by-line coding with their data that help spark ideas and move to a deeper analytical analysis. Students are asked to question the data and ask what is happening with this piece of data. Students are taught to use short, simple names for their codes and use gerunds, if possible, to encourage thinking of processes. Next students make a shared list of codes from all the students' codes that they think fit the data and are significant. Students' memo writing helps them generate useful codes. After students finish one or two exercises together, then they can have confidence to engage in comparative analyses of codes from different interviews. Memo writing is a critical step to help students develop analytic categories.

Charmaz (2015, p. 1618) encouraged students to ask questions like:

- What might their code or category assume?
- Under what conditions is the category discernible?
- Might it be part of a larger process?
- How does a code or category stand up when compared with more data?

Other Faculty's Grounded Theory Teaching Approaches

Hesse-Biber (2007) described two exercises that she has used in teaching undergraduate students. In the first exercise she divided her class into four groups and distributed an interview she had conducted in four segments. Each student individually started open coding of the first segment of the interview. Once finished, students discussed their codes as a group. Hesse-Biber (2007, p. 315) asked the students the following questions:

- What did you decide to code? Did you highlight similar portions of the text?
- Did you assign similar codes? If they were different, talk about your different interpretations.
- What is your overall interpretation of what the respondent is saying in this response? Does the group agree or disagree?

This process was repeated for all four segments of the interview. Then the class reviewed the results it generated and hypothesized about the theory.

Hesse-Biber (2007) described a second assignment she uses with her undergraduate students. Each student is asked to do an interview, record it, transcribe, and analyze it using the grounded theory approach. Students are required to generate at least one theme from their interview that resulted from their open coding process. Next the student hypothesizes what theory could be generated.

Gynnild (2011) attended Glaser's troubleshooting seminars and is a fellow of the Grounded Theory Institute. Gynnild described the principles of teaching by a seminar approach as applied by Glaser as a teacher. Focused presence is the first principle which includes the faculty member's sensitivity and responses to what is going on in the seminar. It is concerned with being present to others and empathetic awareness. Explicitness is a second principle for teaching grounded theory. A seminar leader needs to encourage novice researchers to have trust in the method for them to have confidence in their ability to analyze data. For the faculty member, Glaser stressed to be relaxed, flexible, and in control of the situation. A faculty member should use extensive illustrations of grounded theory studies to help with explicitness. Full acceptance is the third principle where the seminar leader demonstrates genuine curiosity in the participants' work without being judgmental. Deliberate detachment of personal, political, and other presuppositions is required of a seminar leader. The last principle is the principle of vigor. A professor needs to be passionate about teaching grounded theory.

Holton (2019) first attended one of Glaser's 3-day troubleshooting seminars as a PhD student in management and attended several of Glaser's international troubleshooting seminars. Holton now offers her own seminars and was the first editor of the *Grounded Theory Review*. Holton learned that experiential, collaborative learning is at the heart of Glaser's condensed 3-day seminar approach which she in turn teaches novice researchers. She described Glaser's overall approach in the seminar as coaching rather than lecturing.

Simmons (2022; 2024) reflected on his experiences in teaching grounded theory methodology to doctoral students. Simmons explained that in teaching students, faculty need to stress that learning grounded theory is an incremental, recursive process. Also, faculty need to attend to students' emotions such as fear and motivation as they struggle with analysis. Simmons talked about cultivating skill traits like teaching students to be patient and deal with ambiguity and "not knowing" as they analyze grounded theory data. Faculty need to help students minimize preconceptions and guide them to let concepts emerge from data. Simmons assigns a set of Glaser's books for students to read. Learning by doing is essential (Simmons, 2022). Students need to be involved in data collecting, coding, conceptualizing, and identifying core variables. Simmons shared with students some examples of core variables from published literature. Faculty need to caution students to avoid immediately going to established concepts from their specific professional practice and those in the literature. Concepts need to come from data and developing grounded theory. Concepts need to have grab and imagery. Conceptual coding moves students from description to theoretical level and to identify relationships in the data. The critical importance of memo writing and sorting a memo bank is stressed. Simmons directs students to Glaser's theoretical coding families to help in developing a grounded theory.

In the *Grounded Theory Review* White et al. (2024) published an exemplar protocol for a classic Glaserian grounded theory study to help novice researchers. This well-constructed protocol has been approved by an ethics review board. The aim of the protocol is to develop a grounded theory about the primary concerns and behaviors of spousal caregivers who have lost their partners to Parkinson's disease. The following aspects are included under methodology in the protocol: Study design, sampling strategy and size, recruitment, data collection and analysis, and theory development. White et al.'s protocol can be used by faculty in teaching grounded theory to provide a specific example for their students.

My Teaching Strategies

I base my teaching strategies and exercises for my students on the data from my two grounded theory studies. The first study was entitled Teetering on the Edge: A Grounded Theory of Postpartum Depression (Beck, 1993). The second study was entitled Releasing the Pause Button: Mothering Twins During the First Year of Life (Beck, 2002). In this chapter I have chosen this second grounded theory study for examples. In the earlier chapter on Glaserian grounded theory, I briefly described this grounded theory. Now I will continue with it to illustrate some teaching approaches I use with my students.

First, I have my students read the reprint of this study to provide the overall context for the data analysis exercises. In Table 10.1, there is an exercise I use to introduce my students to the beginning steps of Glaser's grounded theory method. It is an excerpt from an interview I conducted with one of the mothers of twins who participated in my research. Students will individually code this interview transcript and then as a class they will share their open codes with each other and compare their coding decisions. In Table 10.2, I have provided my open codes for this excerpt for the faculty and for students who want to check their answers.

The second exercise involves students reading a list of selected open codes from my mothering multiples grounded theory study. Next I ask them individually to begin clustering these codes by constantly comparing and collapsing them into clusters or groupings. Table 10.3 includes a list of selected open codes and Table 10.4 illustrates a beginning clustering of those codes.

TABLE 10.1 Excerpt from Mothering Multiples Interview

I think once they were born, you are really excited beforehand. But once you come home it's a quick reality. I was barely holding my head above water. It was tough and I found that I had to figure it out. I would try to let one baby sleep. I would just nurse him, just fall asleep and the next one would be up. So, I had to learn when one wakes up, after you are done feeding that one, get the next one up. I had to learn to get them on the same schedule as best as I could and that helped me.

The first 4 weeks were kind of in a way kind of a blur because it really was. Basically all I was doing was feeding and changing one baby and then feeding and changing the diaper of the other one. Then the cycle would start again. That was all day and night long. I would try and squeeze in a meal and try to squeeze in a shower and in the afternoon sometimes, I would try and nap for a little bit. In the morning it was like in the evening in many ways. The whole day was sort of the same because they only slept for like 2 ½ hours. It was like being a servant to two very demanding people They weren't really giving anything back then. It definitely was a blur. But then came 3 months and they sort of slept through the night and it was a huge, huge difference. I became like a normal person again.

So, I would say for me the first 3 months you're barely cutting it. I have to say one blessing I did have was some women from a group I'm involved in had women at my baby shower sign up for meals and they brought me dinner for 2 months cause there is just no time to cook. There is no time to clean. There is no time for anything. That's what it is like. Things that were important before would have been my house, vacuuming or whatever. You can't do it. I would cry sometimes because you just can't do it. You have to let it go.

It is a self-sacrifice completely. I'll tell you the first thing I did is when they were 3 months old, I decided to go to the mother of multiples meeting and I kept praying that morning for the strength to get there. Struggling with one screaming and I'm trying to get ready. I thought to myself, I said, 'You know Lord this better be worth it;. And it was. First, I thought, 'How am I going to do this?' I kept seeing moms coming with their strollers and I thought, 'Wow I can do this, I can do this'. That's been a plus. It was just getting out there the first time. Now I look forward to it because I always come home with something even if it's a small nugget. I came home with something. So that was the only time that I really adventured out maybe in 2 months.

There is light at the end of the tunnel. Just push through those first 3 months. It is going to get easier. You will survive. I needed to be organized. Just get everything I needed organized or prepared ahead of time. Take those few minutes when they're happy or doing something on their own when I can pack and get all of it ready even the night before sometimes. Like the morning sometimes when I go to the twins group meetings and need to be there at 10am. Then I make sure that I have the diaper bag packed and I just take any few minutes I have when they don't need my time to get organized and prepared. Get it all out in the car and then I get them last.

I have this ritual of doing everything at night like organizing their bottles and making their meals. Setting up their meals so that when they are hungry, I just go and get it and come back. That way I don't have to fool around. I wash everything and have it all set up and make sure that all the diapers and everything are all stacked. Everything is right there so that I am not running anywhere to find it. Make sure that the diaper bag is full at all times.

(Continued)

TABLE 10.1 (Continued)

The first 3 months I had this schedule on a little piece of paper that you put up on the computer telling me when they ate and about the diaper changes. I knew that was part of helping how much they did those things. Then I would also schedule when they slept. How much they drank during the day when they ate. Now it's very easy, but back then they weren't always easy during the day. They were eating several times a day or more. So, I kept track of when I fed them every day. That is what helped me because I would forget. There was no way I could keep track of it all. So, I have a little sheet so I could keep track of everything.

Yes, being organized is an important part. Also letting things go like saying I can't get to that extra load of laundry. The idea of not being perfect. People couldn't stress that to me enough. It finally sunk in after a couple of months that not everything is going to be perfect and that was okay as long as I was doing my best all the time. I feel like even when I'm overtired and the baby tends to cry a little bit more demandingly and if it takes me an extra minute or two, I just try to tell myself I'm doing the best for them that I can. Prioritizing is also important.

TABLE 10.2 Excerpt from Mothering Multiples Interview with Open Codes

I think once they were born, you are really excited beforehand. But once you come home it's a quick reality. I was barely holding my head above water. It was tough and found that I	Barely holding on
had to figure it out. I would try to let one baby sleep. I would just nurse him, just fall asleep and the next one would be up. So, I had to learn when one wakes up, after you are done	Figuring it out
feeding that one, get the next one up. I had to learn to get them on the same schedule as best as I could and that helped me.	Getting on the same schedule
The first 4 weeks were kind of in a way kind of a blur because it	Blurring
really way. Basically, all I was doing was feeding and changing one baby and then feeding and changing the diaper of the other	Repeating cycle
one. Then the cycle would start again. That was all day and night long. I would try and squeeze in a meal and try to squeeze	Squeezing in
in a shower and in the afternoon sometimes, I would try and nap for a little bit. In the morning it was like in the evening in many ways. The whole day was sort of the same because they only slept for like 2 ½ hours. It was like being a servant to two very	Being a servant
demanding people. They weren't really giving anything back then. It definitely was a blur. But then came 3 months and they sort of slept through the night and it was a huge, huge difference.	Sleeping through the night
I became like a normal person again.	Feeling normal again
So, I would say for me the first 3 months you're barely cutting it.	Barely cutting it
I have to say one blessing I did have was some women from a group I'm involved in has women at my baby shower sign up for	Relying on others
meals and they brought me dinner for 2 months cause there is just no time to cook. There is no time to clean. There is no time	Lack of time
for anything. Things that were important before would have been my house, vacuuming or whatever. You can't do it. I would	Lack of standards
cry sometimes because you just can't do it. You have to let it go.	Letting go

(*Continued*)

TABLE 10.2 (Continued)

It is a self-sacrifice completely. Ill tell you the first time I did is when they were 3 months old, I decided to go to the mother of multiples meeting and I kept praying that morning for the strength to get there. Struggling with the screaming and I'm trying to ger ready. I thought to myself, I said 'You know Lord this better be worth it;, And it was. First, I thought, 'How am I going to do this?' I kept seeing moms coming with their strollers and I thoughts, 'Wow I can do this, I can do this', That's been a plus. It was just getting out there for the first time. Now I look forward to it because I always come home with something ever if it's a small nugget. I came home with something. So that was the only time that I really adventured out maybe in 2 months.	Self-sacrificing Attending multiple meetings Praying for strength Struggling Getting out Adventuring out
There is light at the end of the tunnel. Just push through those first 3 months. It is going to get easier. You will survive. I needed to be organized. Just get everything I needed organized or prepared ahead of time. Take those few minutes when they're happy or doing something on their own when I can pack and get all of it ready even the night before sometimes Like the morning sometimes when I go to the twins group meetings and need to be there at 10am. Then I make sure that I have the diaper bag packed and I just take any few minutes I have when they don't need my time to get organized and prepared. Get it all out in the car and then I get them last.	Pushing through Getting easier Surviving Organizing Planning ahead Preparing
I have this ritual of doing everything at night like organizing their bottles and making their meals. Setting up their meals so that when they are hungry, I just go and get it and come back. That wat I don't have to fool around. I was everything and have it all set up and make sure that all the diapers and everything are all stacked. Everything is right there so that I am not running anywhere to find it. Make sure that the diaper bag is full at all times.	Getting on a routine Making sure
The first 3 months I had this schedule on a little piece of paper that you put up on the computer telling me when they are and about the diaper changed. I knew that was part of helping how much they did those things. Then I would also schedule when they slept. How much they drank during the say when they are. Now its very easy, but back them they weren't always easy during the day. They were eating several times a day or more. So, I kept track of when I fed them every day. That is what helped me because I would forget. There was no way I could keep track of it all. So, I have a little sheet so I could keep track of everything.	Scheduling Keeping track

(Continued)

TABLE 10.2 (Continued)

Yes, being organized it an important part. Also, letting things go like saying I can't get to that extra load of laundry. The idea of not being perfect. People couldn't stress that to me enough. It finally sunk in after a couple of months that not everything is going to be perfect and that was okay as long as I was doing my best all time. I feel like even when I'm overtired and the baby tends to cry a little but more demandingly and it takes me an extra minute or two, I just try to tell myself I'm doing the best for them that I can. Prioritizing is also important.	Being organized Letting things go Exhausting Just doing your best Demanding Prioritizing

TABLE 10.3 Selected In Vivo Codes from Mothering Multiples Study

- Getting regime down
- Going with the flow
- Attending multiples meetings
- Nursing every hour
- Feeling like a milk factory
- Constantly busy
- On hold
- Lacking time for anything else
- Just doing what you can
- Time consuming
- Getting through the day
- Surviving the day
- Exhausting
- Being so tired
- Limiting social life
- Being housebound
- Relinquishing
- Unrelenting
- Non-stop
- Ceaseless
- Unraveling
- Untangling
- Becoming acclimated
- Becoming accustomed
- Flip flopping
- Swapping
- Not stopping living
- Planning
- Mobilizing a team
- Protective remembering
- Blurring
- Getting out
- Being tied down
- Ordeal
- Overwhelming
- Not eating
- Repeating cycle
- Feeling secluded
- Very confining
- Lacking outside connection
- Mentally preparing
- Year out of your life
- Dividing your attention
- Changing plans
- Relying on others
- Demanding
- Going by the wayside
- Pumping
- Appreciating the disabled
- Enlisting help
- Doing your best
- Shifting priorities
- Getting easier
- Becoming manageable
- Prying
- Organizing
- Getting on a routine
- Getting on a schedule
- Canceling plans
- Scheduling
- Not accomplishing tasks
- Letting things go
- Praying to survive
- Getting twins on the same schedule
- Marshaling help
- Tailoring

(Continued)

TABLE 10.3 (Continued)

• Maneuvering	• Physically demanding
• Embarking	• Sleep depriving
• Scaling down	• Enjoying twins
• Pruning	• Strategizing nap times
• Paring	• Making feeding times similar
• In undated	• Weaning
• Submerged	• Attempting nursing twins at same time
• Swamped	• Keeping our sanity
• Keeping afloat	• Staying sane
• Lowering standards	• Doing what works for you
• Prioritizing	

TABLE 10.4 Beginning Clustering of In Vivo Codes from Mothering Multiples Study

• Hanging on	• Self-sacrifice
• Pushing through	• Self-surrender
• Barely cutting it	• Life on hold
• Keeping afloat	• Hitting pause button
• Getting through the day	• Canceling plans
• Surviving the day	
	• Physically demanding
• Blurring	• Draining
• Dulling memory	• Overwhelming
• Protective remembering	• Swamped
	• Inundated
• Confining	• Relentless
• Feeling secluded	• Ceaseless
• Lacking outside connections	
• Being house bound	
• Being tied down	
• Limiting social life	

End-of-Chapter Student Activities

1 This is a discipline-specific activity. Using your discipline's primary data-base, such as ERIC for education, or PsycINFO for psychology, conduct a search for grounded theory studies published in the last 5 years.

   a How many grounded theory studies were published?

   b What specific grounded theory approach was published most often in your discipline?

   c Which grounded theory approach was published the least in your discipline?

   d Share your results with your classmates.

2 In a second student activity, students can choose one of the grounded theory approaches they learned in this textbook such as constructivist grounded theory. Conduct a cross-disciplinary search of databases for the past 5 years for studies that used this grounded theory methodology.

a How many grounded theory studies using this specific approach did you locate?

b In which discipline did researchers use this specific grounded theory approach most often?

c In which discipline did researchers use this specific grounded theory approach the least often?

3 In this student activity only ProQuest dissertation abstracts are searched for the past 5 years. The focus will be on new PhD scholars to learn how often grounded theory was chosen for their dissertations. The student can also search for what grounded theory approach was used most often in these recent dissertations. In what disciplines did the PhD students seem to be choosing grounded theory most often for their dissertations?

References

Beck, C. T. (1993). Teetering on the edge: A substantive theory of postpartum depression. *Nursing Research*, 42, 42–48.

Beck, C. T. (2002). Releasing the pause button: Mothering twins during the first year of life. *Qualitative Health Research*, 12, 593–608. https://doi.org/10.1177/104973202129120124

Charmaz, K. (2015). Teaching theory construction with initial grounded theory tools: A reflection on lessons and learning. *Qualitative Health Research*, 25(12), 1610–1622.

Glaser, B. G. (1998). *Doing grounded theory: Issues and discussions*. Sociology Press.

Glaser, B. G. (2016). *The cry for hope: Preserving autonomy doing GT research*. Sociology Press.

Gynnild, A. (2011). Atmosphering for conceptual discovery. In V. B. Martin & A. Gynnild (Eds.), (pp. 31–49). *Grounded theory: The philosophy, method, and work of Barney Glaser*. Brown Waler Press.

Hesse-Biber, S. (2007). Teaching grounded theory. In A. Bryant & K. Charmaz (Eds.), *Sage handbook of grounded theory* (pp. 311–338). Sage.

Holton, J. A. (2019). Teaching and learning grounded theory methodology: The seminar approach. In A. Bryant & K. Charmaz (Eds.), *The Sage handbook of current developments in grounded theory* (pp. 415–440) Sage.

Simmons, O. E. (2022). *Experiencing grounded theory: A comprehensive guide to learning, doing, mentoring, teaching, and applying grounded theory*. Brown Walker Press.

Simmons, O. E. (2024). "Let the fear go and trust the process"-experiencing grounded theory over a lifetime. *Forum: Qualitative Social Research*, 25(2), Article 8. https://doi.org/10.17169/fqs-25.2.4226

Stern, P. N. (1994). Eroding grounded theory. In J. M. Morse (Ed.), *Critical issues in qualitative research methods* (pp. 212–223). Sage.

White, D. R., White, T. A., & Vander Linden, K. L. (2024). Exploring caregiver grief: A Glaserian (classic) grounded theory protocol. *Grounded Theory Review*, 23(2), 43–59.

11
FUTURE OF GROUNDED THEORY

In this final chapter I offer some future paths grounded theorists can consider following. These paths include freeing Glaser's grounded theory approach from its positivist roots, modifying grounded theory, using social media sources, conducting quantitative grounded theory, formal grounded theory, or grounded theory with mixed methods, and addressing positionality.

Researchers conducting grounded theory studies are fortunate to have both the first- and second-generation approaches to choose from. The bloodline of grounded theory provides alternate choices depending upon the research question being investigated. It is hoped that this book can help researchers decide the grounded theory approach that best matches the purpose of their study so that their desired outcome is the one they hoped for.

For a researcher who wants to conduct a classic Glaserian grounded theory, why can't that researcher modify the epistemological foundation of Glaser's method from positivism to constructivism? A researcher could then co-construct the data and analysis with the participants to help identify the basic problem and process used to resolve that problem. The researcher would not be a passive observer. Reflexivity could then become an important aspect of the modified Glaserian grounded theory approach. Glaser (2005) himself stressed "whether grounded theory takes on the mantle for the moment of prepositivist, positivist, postpositivist, postmodernism, naturalism realism, etc., will be dependent its application to the type of data in a specific research" (p. 145). Holton and Walsh (2017) also argued that grounded theory can be used by researchers irrespective of their philosophical positioning. They viewed Glaser's classic grounded theory methodology as epistemologically and ontologically neutral.

DOI: 10.4324/9781032695563-11

Rarely does one see a modified grounded theory in published literature. Hopefully in the future grounded theorists will be motivated to modify their substantive grounded theories. As Glaser and Strauss (1967) emphasized once a grounded theory is published, "the published word is not the final one, but only a pause in the never-ending process of generating theory" (p. 40). Continued modification is appropriate for all the first- and second-generation grounded theory approaches not just for classic grounded theory.

Another area for future grounded theorists to consider is the use of social media sources for data collection and for outlets to widely communicate their findings. Holton and Walsh (2017) stressed that using social media can provide increased scope for theoretical sampling. Urquhart (2023) and Konecki (2019) also call for the use of visual images in grounded theory methodology.

Glaser and Strauss (1967) in the second half of *The Discovery of Grounded Theory: Strategies for Qualitative Research* explained the possibility of doing quantitative grounded theory. Because Glaser found quantitative grounded theory underdeveloped and lagging behind qualitative grounded theory, he devoted an entire book (Glaser, 2008) to teaching researchers how to generate quantitative grounded theory. Glaser hoped to inspire researchers to attempt a quantitative grounded theory study whose purpose would be to generate conceptual theory and not to test or correct theory. Interested grounded theorists can find more information on conducting quantitative grounded theory in Holton and Walsh's (2017) book *Classic Grounded Theory: Applications with Qualitative and Quantitative Data*. They provide practical guidance on conducting grounded theory in management not only with qualitative data but also with quantitative data in a mixed method study. Advancing grounded theory with mixed methods is another path researchers are starting to follow. Creamer's (2022) book provides information for grounded theorists if they choose this path to follow.

Another path researchers can follow is to pay more attention to the development of formal grounded theory in order to extend the application of substantive grounded theory studies across multiple substantive areas. Formal grounded theory is a theory based on the general implications of a core category from a substantive grounded theory (Glaser, 2007). It is an extension of a core category by modifying it based on the constant conceptual comparative method used in a variety of substantive areas. A researcher does not need to have their own core category to start a formal grounded theory study. Researchers can use a core category found in published grounded theory studies conducted by other researchers. Glaser suggested the following uses of formal grounded theory: Deeper understanding that transcends substantive areas of concern, academic uses like teaching, lectures, policy decisions, modification of extant theories since it operates on a higher abstract level, practical applicability, and cumulative theory.

In future grounded theory studies, more researchers need to address their positionality not only when conducting their studies but also when publishing them (Beck, 2024). While not a mainstream practice in published grounded theory studies, the acknowledgment of the researchers' cultural, political, and social contexts can help readers understand the study's results and help assess any potential biases the researchers may have had. A researcher's positionality can affect six fundamental aspects of a study: Topic of the research, epistemology, ontology, methodology, relationship with participants, and communication (Secules et al., 2021).

Charmaz (2021) stressed that the researcher's positionality is crucial in her constructivist grounded theory approach. In their situational analysis, Clarke et al. (2018) also urged researchers using their grounded theory approach to incorporate reflexivity as a component of the research process. Currently positionality statements are seen more often in published constructivist grounded theory studies than in other grounded theory approaches. A couple of examples of published constructivist grounded theory studies where researchers addressed their positionality are Mazursky's (2025) gender expression of transgender youth in out-of-home care and Yao et al.'s (2025) postgraduate nurses' academic growth trajectory.

Researchers' positionality can shape the perspective through which research decisions are made. Martin et al. (2022) argued that researchers' acknowledging their positions within research can aid in disrupting privilege and bias and can lead to promoting social justice in research. When authors included descriptions of their identities in an article, it helps peel back the curtain on their decision-making while conducting their research which would not otherwise be visible to the readers (Zamzow, 2023). Researchers, however, need to be able to determine how much of their positionality they wish to disclose. There can be personal and professional risks in revealing identities (Oswald, 2024).

Reflexivity goes hand in hand with positionality. It helps in developing transparency in decision-making in the research process. Reflexivity is the process of the researchers' critical self-reflection about their own experiences, biases, preferences, preconceptions, and beliefs that could impact their decisions in conducting a grounded theory study no matter which grounded theory approach is used. Keeping reflexive diaries and self-reflexive memos are two strategies grounded theorists can use. There are some published strategies to help researchers address reflexivity and write positionality statements. One example is Reyes' (2020) ethnographic toolkit to aid researchers in identifying their multiple social positions during the research process. Mruck and Mey (2019) offer another example, research interviews, at the start of a research project to help with reflexivity. These interviews are with team members where they interview each other about their emotions and pre-assumptions regarding the topic of the study.

Charmaz (2017; 2025) emphasized that grounded theory has the potential to make change in the world for the better. In order to help accomplish this, grounded theorists need to enhance the impact of their findings by communicating them in a way that translates them for practical applications. Birk and Mills (2023) offered five general factors that researchers can consider when communicating their grounded theory through publishing or orally presenting their results:

- Identify the audience.
- Determine what level of analytical detail is needed.
- Present the grounded theory as a whole.
- Make specific and useful recommendations.
- Match the style of writing to the chosen audience.

These suggestions mirror Glaser's (1978) wish that when researchers report a grounded theory study, it includes an application for their discipline's practice with recommendations. Since this book is for health and social science researchers, this final recommendation for improving each of our discipline's practice is especially relevant.

References

Beck, C. T. (2024). Perspectives on positionality statements in scholarly discourse. *Journal of Obstetric, Gynecologic, and Neonatal Nursing, 53*(6), 581–584. https://doi.org/10.1016/j.jogn.2024.09.010

Birk, M., & Mills, J. (2023). *Grounded theory: A practical guide*. Sage.

Charmaz, K. (2017). The power of constructivist grounded theory for critical inquiry. *Qualitative Inquiry, 23*(1), 34–35. https://doi.org/10.1177/1077800416657105

Charmaz, K. (2021). The genesis, grounds, and growth of constructivist grounded theory in J. M. Morse, B. J. Bowers, K. Charmaz, A. E. Clarke, J. Corbin, & C. J. Porr with P. N. Stern (Eds.), *Developing grounded theory: The second generation revisited*. (pp. 153–187). Routledge.

Charmaz, K. (2025). *Constructing grounded theory* (3rd ed.). Sage.

Clarke, A. E., Friese, C., & Washburn, R. (2018). *Situational analysis: Grounded theory after the interpretive turn* (2nd ed.). Sage.

Creamer, E. G. (2022). *Advancing grounded theory with mixed methods*. Routledge.

Glaser, B. G. (1978). *Theoretical sensitivity: Advances in the methodology of grounded theory*. Sociology Press.

Glaser, B. G. (2005). *The grounded theory perspective III: Theoretical coding*. Sociology Press.

Glaser, B. G. (2007). *Doing formal grounded theory: A proposal*. Sociology Press.

Glaser, B. G. (2008). *Doing quantitative grounded theory*. Sociology Press.

Glaser, B. G., & Strauss, A. (1967). *The discovery of grounded theory: Strategies for qualitative research*. Aldine de Gruyter.

Holton, J. A., & Walsh, I. (2017). *Classic grounded theory: Applications with qualitative & quantitative data*. Sage.

Konecki, K. T. (2019). Visual images and grounded theory methodology. In A. Bryant & K. Charmaz (Eds.), *The SAGE handbook of current developments in grounded theory* (pp. 352–373). Sage.

Martin, J. P., Desing, R., & Borrego, M. (2022). Positionality statements are just the tip of the iceberg: Moving towards a reflexive process. *Journal of Women and Minorities in Science and Engineering*, *28*(4), v–vii. http://dx.doi.org/10.1615/JWomenMinorScienEng.2022044277

Mazursky, N. (2025). Exploring gender expression: Experiences of transgender youth in out-of-home care. *Child Abuse & Neglect*, *160*, 107167. https://doi.org/10.1016/j.chiabu.2024.107167

Mruck, K., & Mey, G. (2019). Grounded theory methodology and self-reflexivity in the qualitative process. In A. Bryant & K. Charmaz (Eds.), *The SAGE handbook of current developments in grounded theory* (pp. 470–496). Sage.

Oswald, R. (2024). Positionality statements should not force us to 'out' ourselves. *Nature Human Behaviour*, *8*(2), Article 185. https://doi.org/10.1038/s41562-023-01812-5

Reyes, V. (2020). Ethnographic toolkit: Strategic positionality and researchers' visible and invisible tools in field research. *Ethnography*, *21*(2), 220–240. https://doi.org/10.1177/1466138118805121

Secules, S., McCall, C., Mejia, J. A., Beebe, C., Masters, A. S., Sánchez-Peña, M. L., & Svyantek, M. (2021). Positionality practices and dimensions of impact on equity research: A collaborative inquiry and call to the community. *Journal of Engineering Education*, *110*(1), 19–43. https://doi.org/10.1002/jee.20377

Urquhart, C. (2023). *Grounded theory for qualitative research*. Sage.

Yao, H., Xie, C., Luo, M., & Luo, Y. (2025). "A level-breaking adventure game": A grounded theory study of postgraduate nurses' academic growth trajectory. *Nurse Education Today*, *146*, 106520. https://doi.org/10.1016/j.nedt.2024.106520

Zamzow, R. (2023). Scientists clash over positionality statements. *Science*, *382*(6670), 501. https://doi.org/10.1126/science.adm6801

INDEX

Note: Page references with *Italics* refer to figures, **bold** refer to tables.